THE
SKINCARE
HOAX

THE
SKINCARE HOAX

How You're Being Tricked into Buying Lotions, Potions & Wrinkle Cream

FAYNE L. FREY, MD
board-certified dermatologist and skincare consultant

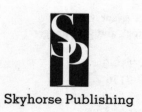

Skyhorse Publishing

WARNING

What I'm about to reveal will be completely contrary to what you believe about skin, about skincare, and about yourself. The opinions expressed in this book are based on my chemistry background and my experience with skincare formulation, along with my knowledge of medical research and thirty years' experience as a dermatologist. The material I provide is designed to offer helpful information on the subject matters discussed and is not, in any way, meant to be used to diagnose or treat any medical condition. To do so, consult your own physician or medical provider.

Now I'm ready to tell the truth, the whole truth, and nothing but the truth. Please keep an open mind and get ready to be blown away.

Skyhorse Publishing books may be purchased in bulk at special discounts for sales promotion, corporate gifts, fund-raising, or educational purposes. Special editions can also be created to specifications. For details, contact the Special Sales Department, Skyhorse Publishing, 307 West 36th Street, 11th Floor, New York, NY 10018 or info@skyhorsepublishing.com.

Skyhorse® and Skyhorse Publishing® are registered trademarks of Skyhorse Publishing, Inc.®, a Delaware corporation.

Visit our website at www.skyhorsepublishing.com.

10 9 8 7 6 5 4 3 2 1

Library of Congress Cataloging-in-Publication Data is available on file.

Jacket design by David Ter-Avanesyan
Jacket images by Shutterstock and gettyimages

Print ISBN: 978-1-5107-7155-0
Ebook ISBN: 978-1-5107-7156-7

Printed in the United States of America

To every woman who was told she needed a beauty fix . . .
and walked away.

Contents

Foreword

This gem of a book, written by well-known dermatologist Fayne L. Frey, MD, exposes some well-kept secrets of the beauty industry, such as repurposing the exact same ingredients into differently sized and colored jars and tubes. Each of these products is designed to target a different market, for instance, face, body, eyes, or kids. Each category has a different price point (and a widely varying price per pound). It's as if the industry believes that we believe that the skin of our eyes is worth much more than the skin elsewhere on our bodies.

The book also reveals how "big marketing" is used to sell us on the idea that we must use certain products in order to be worthy in our beauty-conscious society. You know the spiel: Use this product to look younger, more beautiful, more alluring. The problem is that this type of messaging works. The half-trillion-dollar beauty industry is a tribute to the marketing genius that gets us to spend a lot of our hard-earned money on products that don't come close to delivering what we thought they were promising.

What I really love about this book is that the author does not shy away from naming names. That's how I learned that my old faithful moisturizer is not on her list of most effective moisturizers. She should know; she has used a device to measure the water content of her patients' skin after using different products.

She also doesn't dumb things down. She explains the science, provides the references, and encourages us to actually learn what is in the stuff that we liberally smear all over our bodies, sometimes multiple times a day.

Dr. Frey warns us at the beginning of the book that she is going to tell the truth, the whole truth, and nothing but the truth—and she does. This book is a valuable resource for anyone who uses beauty products on a regular basis—and that includes most of us. I highly recommend that you get a copy and keep it near your computer to consult the next time you go online to replenish your products.

Patricia Salber, MD
founder and editor-in-chief,
The Doctor Weighs In

Introduction

Almost two decades ago, a friendly woman from Philadelphia (I'll call her Lisa, not her real name) visited my office in West Nyack, New York. She came in for a first-visit evaluation. She walked into my office carrying a sizable bag of skincare products and dumped bottles and tubes all over my desk.

She said, "Dr. Frey, everything I put on my face makes me break out."

I picked up one of the bottles and read the ingredients. Lisa had no way of knowing that in college I was a chemistry buff. I was curious—you might even say obsessed—about the ingredients in skincare products. Chemical names fascinated me. I wanted to know what they were and how they worked. That was my nerdy secret.

Lisa sat quietly while I looked through her pile of products. I saw all kinds of red flags: octyl stearate, isopropyl myristate, acetylated lanolin alcohol, cocoa butter, and more. Finally, I said, "From what I know of the research, you shouldn't use these. Many of these products have ingredients that might cause you to break out."

She tapped the arm of her chair and burst out, "I went to an Ivy League school, and I have a corner office at my firm. I consider myself a fairly bright woman. How am I supposed to know what to use?"

That's when it dawned on me. Every single day, women stare at that wall of skincare products in their local pharmacy or surf online, with no idea what to choose. All they see is marketing on the front label that convinces them they're not adequate the way they are. Where do people go to find solid, scientific information about what to buy?

That conversation with Lisa stayed with me all day. I went home that evening and put together an idea for an online skincare product selector that would help women make informed decisions. By filling in a few criteria, the program would list the products that fit their personal preferences and their specific concerns. After many months of research and design, I hired a computer programmer to put the selector on my website, FryFace.com, and introduced it to several of my acne and eczema patients. In my mind, the project was complete.

A few weeks later, I received a call from Z100, a New York radio station. They told me my website was trending. I wasn't exactly sure what that meant, but they assured me trending is a good thing. They asked to feature my Product Selector on their "What's Trending" segment of *Elvis Duran and the Morning Show.*

The website was free to everyone, so why not? I said, "Sure."

That opened the floodgates. I got a call from CBS TV asking, "Are you Dr. Frey from FryFace.com?" After I confirmed my identity, they asked, "Do you sell products? Do you represent a manufacturer?" I answered "no" to both questions.

They then asked me if I would participate as a medical expert for an exposé on the safety of over-the-counter skincare products. They wanted facts. They came to my office and filmed for several hours. I talked about a day cream being the same as a night cream, except day cream has sunscreen. I revealed that eye cream is simply a formulated moisturizer in a smaller tube. The only thing special about eye cream is the price.

I received a call from a writer at *USA Today*. "Are you Dr. Frey from FryFace.com?" Once again, I confirmed my identity. "Do you sell products? Do you represent a manufacturer?"

When I said no, they asked if I'd help with an article about the efficacy of "anti-wrinkle creams." Again, they wanted facts.

Speaking invitations flooded my inbox. One of my favorite openers is, "If you work the night shift, should you wear day cream?" to show how ludicrous some of these claims are. Around the same time, I wrote an op-ed piece for NBC News. I received invitations to be a contributor for *The Doctor Weighs In*, *50Plus-Today*, and *Reader's Digest* online magazine, in addition to medical expert requests to consult for articles in HuffPost, Business Insider, Zwivel, LifeHacker, and many other online media outlets.

Requests came in from both readers and the media for me to write a book. I have a thriving dermatology practice where I specialize in skin cancer. I didn't know how I'd find the time for such a massive project, so I put off the book idea. With encouragement from family, friends, and patients, I eventually got that inner urge and decided to go for it.

So, here we are at the meeting of my passion for truth, my drive to empower women with information, and my perverse tendency to mock the system. Seriously, sometimes this stuff gets so absurd, all you can do is laugh.

Before we begin, I'd like to emphasize that I have no financial interest in any product that I recommend, nor do I represent any particular skincare manufacturer. My hope is that this book will empower women around the globe to turn away from the "I'm not good enough" marketing messages they see hundreds of times each day and realize how truly awesome they already are.

—Fayne L. Frey, MD

CHAPTER 1

Are You Being Served or Sold?

Why do accomplished, intelligent women spend so much money on skincare products that don't work? Why do they put so much energy into looking a certain way? These questions hover in the back of my mind every day in my dermatology practice.

I see women spend $300 for a one-ounce jar of face cream, use it for a few months, then realize they don't see results. So, they purchase a new product at $500 an ounce. Once again, they come to the same conclusion: it's not working. They search again and purchase something else. My heart goes out to them. I know what they are actually buying, and it isn't what they think.

Too many patients arrive at my office in a state of anxiety because they found a fine line on their forehead. They have no concerns about cancer. They just want that little wrinkle to go away.

Why?

Why is it that every newsflash of some so-called break-through discovery has millions of already-fabulous women lining up to spend money they may or may not have to reach for a goal they never seem to attain? The answer lies within a $500 billion cosmetic industry that wants to sell products. It lies within a sector of cosmetics called the skincare industry.

Do these products truly support healthy skin? The answer is in the science, but how do those scientific findings apply to the claims of specific creams, gels, and lotions? The answer is not simple or easy. In fact, it's a long and winding road with several detours.

Cosmetics and Advertising

"Cosmetics are not a modern invention. Humans have used various substances to alter their appearance or accentuate their features for at least ten thousand years, and possibly longer."* In ancient Egypt, women used lead-based powder called *kohl* to darken their eyelids. In ancient China, both men and women stained their fingernails various colors to show their social class. Cleopatra is famous for her milk baths she claimed made her skin soft and smooth.**

In modern times, an important element has shaped our global culture: marketing. Cosmetic print ad campaigns have been around for more than a hundred years. In the 1920s, the Sweet Georgia Brown company sold Wonderful Vanishing Cream and Magic Pink Lovin' Cream*** (whatever that means). A company

---

* Jones, "The chemistry of cosmetics."

** Ibid.

*** Vanity Treasures, "Vintage Cosmetic Set/Vintage Cosmetic Sets / Vintage Sample Make-Up Kit / Vintage Sample Make-Up Sample Kits."

called Durney's published ads for Gay Paree Vanishing Cream* to make a woman's skin glow—or so they said.

In the 1950s, television brought a wide-open opportunity for marketing into our homes. Over the next twenty years, the cosmetic industry created an entire cultural mythology that told women what they need for the best-looking face and hair. What started out as catchy commercials in the 1950s became a universal belief system today.

Let's consider shampoo, for example. Ask any woman over seventy what she used to wash her hair as a young girl, and she'll look confused. She'll probably say she can't remember. Then she might say dishwashing liquid, brown soap, or some type of oil. In 1908 *The New York Times* published an article on how to use castile soap—also used for dishes and laundry—to wash hair.**

> *"Ask any woman over seventy what she used to wash her hair as a young girl, and she'll look confused."*

A 1920s radio ad for Luster-Cream Shampoo promised that shampooing would increase sex appeal. In 1952 a TV commercial for Drene shampoo showed a teenager getting ready for a date by washing his hair.*** By the 1970s Farrah Fawcett commercials told consumers that shampooing less than several times a week was unhealthy.****

What about the instructions on many shampoo bottles that say, "Lather, Rinse, Repeat"? Why repeat? There are no proven

---

* Ralph's Closet, "Derny's Gay Paree Vanishing Cream Small Bottle Boudoir Vanity Piece 1920s Cosmetics Flapper Logo."

** Hairstory.com, "The History of Shampoo."

*** Sherrow, "Encyclopedia of Hair: A Cultural History," 8.

**** Hairstory.com, "The History of Shampoo."

health benefits to shampooing twice, although repeating the process empties the shampoo bottle twice as fast.

This is just one simplified example of the progression of marketing and myth-building. How many moms today teach their children to wash their hair every time they shower? What started out as an ad campaign turned into a cultural norm.

So, what caused the invention of shampoo? Did soap makers hear about a breakthrough in science showing that people need a special soap for hair, and need to use it almost every day in order to be healthy? Or did a smart copy writer come up with a tantalizing way to sell the product and then double sales by adding one little word to their simple instructions: Repeat?

Unfortunately, most of the time this kind of information is just marketing, pure and simple.

> *"Dozens of beliefs we commonly hold true today were made up more than fifty years ago in an ad campaign."*

Shampoo is only one example. Dozens of beliefs we commonly hold true today were made up more than fifty years ago by someone at a typewriter working up an ad campaign.

Here are just a few of them:

- Dermatologist-tested products are better.
- Women over fifty should use skincare products designed for mature skin.
- Hypoallergenic means you'll never have a reaction to that product.
- The more expensive the product, the better it is.
- Take your makeup off before you go to sleep or you'll get wrinkles. (What you'll actually get is a dirty pillowcase!)
- Sleep on your back to avoid wrinkles.

This is the cosmetics industry—a $500 billion playground so mixed in its messages that the consumer has no idea what is truly helpful and what is simply hype. I sat down to write this book to bring some sense to the nonsense out there—to deliver the facts and tell the truth about what's really helpful and what's glitz and glam. But first, I want to make it clear that, as a dermatologist, I'm here as your advocate, to help you understand what best supports your skin, so you can make informed choices and avoid wasting money on products that don't do what you expect.

If someone wants to use an expensive product that feels creamy and smells great—although it doesn't do much to keep their skin healthy—that's their choice, and I honor that. My primary concern is that they make an informed decision.

More Is Better, or Is It?

Cosmetic companies go to great lengths to convince consumers that without certain essential items in their beauty regimen, they will age faster and look shabby. Ads all too often use pseudoscience to glorify youth and instill a deep longing for a face that doesn't age.

Many women use more than a dozen products every morning while dressing for work. With the average product containing fifteen to fifty different ingredients, she can unknowingly expose herself to an estimated 515 chemicals before breakfast.*

This is totally unnecessary.

I had a client who filled her bathroom counter with dozens of products worth hundreds of dollars, but she rarely used them. She purchased them with good intentions of following certain beauty regimens but felt rushed getting ready for work or was too tired at night. As a result, she failed to follow through. Every time she brushed her teeth, those pretty little bottles and jars

---

* Jones, "The chemistry of cosmetics."

stood like an accusing mob, blaming her for not using expensive products for which she had paid good money.

After learning the truth about those various items, she pushed all of them off the counter and into a garbage bag, except for her basic moisturizer and sunscreen. At her next appointment, she gave me a glowing smile and said, "I feel so liberated. No more guilt!"

The first step in your reality check is to find out whether your current products support healthy skin. Many of these creams feel good, but are they actually good for your skin?

> *"Many of these creams feel good, but are they actually good for your skin?"*

Well-formulated moisturizers optimize how your skin looks and allow it to function at its best. These moisturizers can improve conditions like acne, rosacea, and eczema. Scientific studies also show the health benefits of applying daily sunscreen.* Any product other than sunscreen and moisturizer requires a closer look into how it affects the skin—whether helpful or harmful.

I'm not saying all cosmetics marketing is bad. However, many of these companies create fake problems, so they can offer a solution that sells more products. Sensationalism sells, especially when said in a way that touches the most sensitive emotion in a woman—her longing to look her best. The next few chapters address this issue in more detail, but let's just say the cosmetic industry floods the airwaves with its message that no woman can look good enough without spending more and more and more.

You know that old story about "The Woman Who Lived in a Shoe"? She had to live in a shoe because she spent all her

---

* Halpern, "The Melanoma Letter."

hard-earned cash on expensive skincare products, and she couldn't afford a house. Sadly, too many women fall into that category.

I received validation for this line of thinking when one of my patients, Tracey Damiani, came to my office and told me this story. Tracey is brilliant and delightful . . . and she also worked in the cosmetic industry for decades. She was kind enough to write her story in a letter and give me permission to use it:

I have recently been told about a new site called FryFace.com. All I can say is—it's about time! I am an esthetician and makeup artist who has worked for twenty-five years for almost every high-end cosmetic company.

I remember coming home from my first training seminar. I was in awe of all the new products I had learned about, from "lift serums," "anti-puff eye gel," "sunspot removers," etc.

I was excited to tell my grandfather my new information. Being a chemist for a large makeup company for forty years, he went ingredient by ingredient and explained what they were and how not one product would do what I was trying to convince him of! He said, "Doll, just don't use [harsh] soap as a cleanser and always moisturize."

I thought, *what does he know?* I was nineteen years old and believed every word! I used those fancy products for many years, layering two and three at a time, and guess what . . . now at forty-three I realize he was *right*!

I will never forget my last job, an expensive skincare line. My goal was [to sell] $1,000 a day and I had a great rep. I could sell anything and everything, but I just began to feel bad. Telling these women that a $400.00+ cream was going to change how they looked while I was using an $18 moisturizer and Oil of Olay® cleanser. That was it for me. My sales days were over.

Every person looking for that miracle in a bottle *must* go to this site. It is long overdue in my eyes, easy to navigate, and very informative. So good luck . . . save your money . . .

Gratefully,
Tracey Damiani

To put costs in perspective, many creams come in beautiful little one-ounce jars. An ounce is the amount in a shot glass*. Let's say, you want to save money, so you go to Target or Wal-Mart and pick up one of those jars for $22.99. That seems like a great deal compared to the $300-per-ounce variety. However, when you consider a pound has 16 ounces, that cheaper brand still costs $367.84 a pound. If you pick up some inexpensive eye cream for $17 per half-ounce tube, you're paying $544 per pound. High-end cream at $300 per ounce skyrockets to $4,800 per pound.

It's no wonder the tycoons on *Shark Tank* give earnest attention to someone who comes in with a skincare line. The markups are incredible. Unfortunately, women pay the price—in more ways than one. From the science perspective, more expensive doesn't mean better. Skin isn't impressed by a price tag because what works is actually pretty simple and very affordable.

---

* An ounce, noted as oz, measures the weight of a dry substance. A fluid ounce, represented by fl oz, measures the volume occupied by a liquid. Since a fluid ounce of water weighs approximately 1 ounce, and since water is the ingredient with the highest concentration in the majority of skincare formulations referred to in this book, these units are used interchangeably.

> *"Skin isn't impressed by a price tag because what works is actually pretty simple and very affordable."*

Two essential products that support healthy skin are well-formulated moisturizers and sunscreens. They belong in every bathroom, makeup case, and travel kit.

I recommend products that are effective and have scientifically proven claims on their labels. Fortunately, reputable skincare companies produce many such products. I say *usually* because even effective products sometimes have unscientific words on their labels.

Take, for example, the word *nourishing*. Skin cells that are in contact with moisturizers are dead. It's scientifically impossible to nourish dead tissue. Yet, some great products might have the word *nourishing* in bold letters on their label. That doesn't make the company bad or the product less effective, but the informed consumer knows the word *nourishing* doesn't have any real meaning. They'll look closer at the label to see if the product is worth buying.

On the other hand, many product labels contain word games, tall tales, and unscientific statements. These products might have some benefit for the skin as well-formulated moisturizers. However, their marketing promises youth and beauty in a pretty little jar for as much as $8,400 per pound. They mislead the consumer by creating unrealistic expectations. I'll go into more detail later, but some of their buzzwords are *anti-aging, firming,* and *age-defying,* to name a few.

Unfortunately, many reputable companies sell both types of moisturizers: those marketed appropriately, and others studded with hype. Some will take an excellent moisturizer, package it as an age-defying eye cream, and add a label that creates unrealistic expectations. Products with labels that misinform and overpromise are sold everywhere, in supermarkets, pharmacies, salons, on the Internet, by direct sales, and even in doctors' offices.

Other cosmetics promise to benefit the skin with no science proving they are effective. Most people with healthy skin don't need them. These products might feel good and smell good, and they might be fun to apply, but they don't necessarily benefit skin health. In some cases, they might even cause skin irritation, flaking, and dryness. Some of them are quite costly.

So, how does the consumer tell which products have proven health benefits? Everywhere we look—four thousand to ten thousand times per day, according to Forbes®*—we see ads that fuel our self-doubts and send the subliminal message, "I'm not good enough the way I am." These ads promise that their miracle potion makes you look ten years younger, including a youthful glow and a sparkle in your eye. In other words, the product makes you look like the girl in the ad when even the model doesn't look like the girl in the ad.

> *"Pronouncing individual brands as good or bad doesn't work."*

Calling individual brands good or bad doesn't work. Johnson & Johnson® owns Aveeno® which makes quality moisturizers. They also own Neutrogena® which produces some good moisturizers but also sells a night cream with Retinol (more on the Retinol topic later). Another company, Cerave®, makes effective moisturizers that I recommend to my patients, but Cerave® also sells an eye cream. Both night creams and eye creams are simply moisturizers.

---

* Simpson, "Finding Brand Success In The Digital World."

Most reputable manufacturers cross this line at some point, so this is a product-by-product issue. The only way to be certain about what you're buying is to read the ingredient listing. However, ingredients with long scientific names are of little help to the ordinary person with no science background.

> *"This is a product-by-product issue."*

To be clear, this isn't a question of good companies and bad companies, but rather helpful products, overpromised products, and unnecessary products.

How Skin Actually Works

When most people think of skin, they think about the external surface of the body. However, the skin is much more than an outer covering. It is the largest organ of the body with several functions: detecting sensory information, maintaining body temperature, providing a physical barrier to protect the body, and its most critical function, preventing water loss.*

> *"This skin barrier is amazingly strong and durable."*

This skin barrier is amazingly strong and durable. When you wash up the pots and pans after a big dinner, you use detergent and a scrubber to clean them. When you finish, you rinse your hands, dry them on a towel, and go on with your day. Despite all the hot water and detergent, your hands look the same as before. That's the function of healthy skin. The outermost layer of the

---

* Purnamawati, "The Role of Moisturizers in Addressing Various Kinds of Dermatitis: A Review."

skin called the epidermis has several layers. For our purposes, we're focusing on the top layer where the most mature nonliving, yet

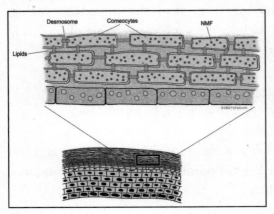

functional, skin cells occur. These cells (corneocytes) are mostly made of the protein keratin. Each cell contains Natural Moisturizing Factor (NMF), which are tiny sponge-like bodies that draw water to the skin surface from below and also from the environment. A fatty lipid layer covers each cell to make the skin virtually water repellent.

Simply stated, the NMF sponges draw in water, and the lipid layer locks it in. Quality moisturizers support the lipid barrier by helping to hold water in.

Healthy skin is in a constant process of renewal. Living skin cells migrate up from the bottom layer of the epidermis toward the outer surface where they eventually become part of the twenty layers of dead cells covering the body. The dead cells have tiny bridges that join them together. Over time, enzymes break down those tiny bridges, which allows old cells to fall away so newer ones can come to the surface.

These enzymes require moisture. Without adequate hydration, the shedding process falters, so the skin looks flaky and feels rough. Quality moisturizers support these enzymes by helping the skin hold on to water. When old cells fall away, the skin feels soft and smooth. That's why I always say the best exfoliant is a good moisturizer.

"That's why I always say the best exfoliant is a good moisturizer."

Some people have special skin conditions where the skin doesn't go through this process efficiently, such as atopic dermatitis or eczema. Because of a defective barrier, areas of their skin become an open door. The skin releases its water into the environment, and the body has the constant stress of germ invaders and chemical intruders. The skin becomes dry and irritated. Whenever any abnormal skin condition persists, if a rash develops, or if symptoms occur such as itching, redness, oozing, or pain, it's time to consult a medical professional.

For the purposes of this work, I'm generally referring to normal healthy skin and how to care for it—commonly known as skincare.

Cosmetics vs. Drugs

When you make a product choice, it's important to know the distinction between a cosmetic and a drug as defined by the US Food and Drug Administration (FDA). Skincare manufacturers are careful to market their wares within the confines of the law because the consequences are huge. Crossing the line can put them out of business.

In 1938, Congress passed a law called the Federal Food, Drug, and Cosmetic Act (FD&C Act.) that defined a cosmetic by its intended use "for cleansing, beautifying, promoting attractiveness, or altering the appearance."* Examples of cosmetics are soaps, shower gels, fragrances, perfumes, lipsticks, fingernail polishes, tanning products, skin moisturizers, eye and facial makeup preparations, shampoos, permanent waves, hair colors, toothpastes, and deodorants.**

---

* [FD&C Act, sec. 201(i)] https://www.fda.gov/cosmetics/cosmetics-laws -regulations/it-cosmetic-drug-or-both-or-it-soap#Definedrug

** FDA, "Are all 'personal care products' regulated as cosmetics?" https://www.fda.gov/industry/fda-basics-industry/are-all-personal-care -products-regulated-cosmetics

Drugs are substances other than food "intended to *affect the structure or any function* of the body of man or other animals"* [Emphasis mine]. Drugs make structural changes and treat conditions. Drug manufacturers go to great expense to acquire FDA premarket approval and prove safety and efficacy before they launch a product. For example, the US regulates sunscreen as a drug because it claims to help prevent sunburn or to decrease the risks of skin cancer and early skin aging caused by the sun.

> *"Drugs make structural changes and treat conditions."*

Some drugs need a prescription, but others—called over-the-counter (OTC) drugs—are available off the shelf. One way to tell if something is a drug is its Drug Facts label.** Similar to the Nutrition Facts label on food packaging, the Drug Facts label has its own requirements. Almost all OTC drugs have this label with few exceptions.

Some products are both cosmetics and drugs, such as dandruff shampoo. The cleansing aspect of the shampoo makes it a cosmetic, and its claim as a dandruff treatment makes it a drug. Look for a Drug Facts label to know whether the product you're looking at is a drug. This is important because knowing the difference between a drug and a cosmetic will affect your buying decisions.

> *"A cosmetic promotes attractiveness and alters the appearance."*

---

* [FD&C Act, sec. 201(i)] https://www.fda.gov/cosmetics/cosmetics-laws-regulations/it-cosmetic-drug-or-both-or-it-soap#Definedrug

** FDA, "OTC Drug Facts Label." https://www.fda.gov/drugs/drug-information-consumers/otc-drug-facts-label

A drug intends to make structural changes and treats or prevents conditions. A cosmetic promotes attractiveness and alters the appearance. Cosmetics don't truly intend to change anything, not permanently, if at all.

Cosmetic manufacturers are well aware they do not have to show proof of their cosmetic claims before they go to market. And, they have a lot of leeway in their marketing and advertising.

If a manufacturer intends for their "anti-aging" cream to change the structure or function of the skin (as in getting rid of wrinkles), that cream must be legally classified as a drug and have premarket FDA approval and proof that it's safe and effective. The vetting process costs millions of dollars before the product gets to market. It's an expensive endeavor that would drastically cut into the profits of a cosmetic manufacturer.

So, you see, cosmetic manufacturers can't intend for their products to change the skin. That's why wrinkle-cream ads promise to "decrease the *appearance* of fine lines" rather than "remove fine lines." *Reducing the appearance* is the legally compliant language for cosmetics. *Remove* is the legally compliant language for a drug. This subtle difference can confuse people who don't know the significance of the words. A cosmetic that claims to remove wrinkles is in violation of federal law.

"A cosmetic that claims to remove wrinkles is in violation of federal law."

The FryFace Rules

Over the years, I've found myself repeating certain facts again and again. Eventually, I made a list of statements I say most often, both when I speak and in print. I call them The FryFace Rules. This simple list provides some general guidelines for when you're standing at that beauty wall in the pharmacy or shopping online.

Rule #1
Science has yet to discover a single product or ingredient that can reverse the aging process.

Rule #2
The most important information on a skincare bottle is the ingredient listing.

Rule #3
By law, over-the-counter cosmetics, including facial moisturizers, cannot intend to change the structure or function of skin or they'd be classified as drugs.

Rule #4
The cost of a skincare product is not a measure of its effectiveness.

Rule #5
The best recipe for healthy, optimal appearing skin is a healthy lifestyle. Magic potions don't exist. If a product seems too good to be true, it probably is.

Rule #6
You are fabulous the way you are. When in doubt, look in the mirror and repeat, "Dear Me, I'm Awesome!"

These simple principles help steer you in the right direction. Knowing the difference between a cosmetic and a drug, you can identify marketing hype that cannot be true. If they were true, the manufacturer would have the Feds on their case.

How can marketing campaigns lead people to believe unproven statements? I'll get into that in more detail in Chapter 6 on page 79, but for now, let's just say, much of this stuff doesn't make sense. Ad campaigns aren't about logic or science. They are all about marketing and sales.

For example, women's magazines are one of the major outlets for cosmetic ads. They depend on their core advertisers to stay in business. If they filled their pages with articles exposing unproven claims and overpromised expectations, they would lose their main income stream. I've seen this firsthand.

A few years back, a popular beauty magazine interviewed me about FryFace.com. I spent a couple of hours teaching the editor about how the skin functions and about skincare ingredients and product formulation. I showed her scientific studies to back up what I told her and dispelled many skincare myths we frequently hear from advertisers, the media, and self-proclaimed "skin experts."

She loved that I was educating consumers about skincare without the hype and that I had no financial interest in any product or particular manufacturer. She loved my mission to educate women to help them select safe, effective, and affordable skincare products. After our interview she told me she planned on running a full spread about FryFace.com.

I was overjoyed. Three days later I received a phone call from the senior health editor from that same publication. She said abruptly, "I'm sorry to inform you, but we must pull the story on FryFace."

Of course, I asked why. I told her she was in a great position to educate thousands of women and cut through the widespread misinformation from the skincare industry.

She simply replied, "I'm so sorry. I have a business to run."

We are at a point in our global culture similar to the Hans Christian Anderson tale "The Emperor's New Clothes."* In the story, crafty swindlers convinced the emperor they could make

---

* Wikipedia contributors, "The Emperor's New Clothes."

him a new suit of clothes only smart and worthy people could see. They told him anyone who couldn't see the suit was foolish. The entire country turned out to see the new clothes, and everyone was afraid to say what they clearly saw: the emperor wore no clothes. Finally, a child blurted out the truth, and the mob chased the charlatans out of town.

The same is true of "anti-aging" serums and lotions that claim to dissolve fine lines and wrinkles to restore more youthful skin. These magic potions cost as much as $500 per ounce or $8,000 per pound. No one dares tell a woman who has invested her time and money that they don't see much difference, certainly not her family and friends. That isn't polite. Besides, she loves the look of those pretty jars reflected in the mirror of her makeup table.

Over the thirty years I've practiced medicine, my passion remains unchanged. I strive to give women information that is true and effective, to point them toward positive lifestyle choices and help them feel better about themselves.

I recently had a kind, accomplished, curvy woman come into my office. As with many of my patients, I asked her to look in the mirror and say, "Dear Me, I'm Awesome!"

She burst into tears.

Yes, this overweight woman had her challenges. But slender twenty-year-old women do the same thing in my office. So do thirty-year-olds, and women in their forties, on up through every age range, regardless of their physical appearance. How many women around the world can look into a mirror and say those words without feeling like a fraud? Far too few.

It's time for someone to speak up about how the beauty industry affects the lives of amazing, strong, and wonderful women. With accurate information and a little perspective, women can feel empowered and beautiful at any age. That's my message. Now let's take a look at the details.

CHAPTER 2

Marketing: A Multi-Billion Dollar Industry of Illusion

Products that support skin health and also have transparent marketing are at the sweet spot for making a solid buying decision. When either the benefits or the marketing goes awry, women likely choose products based on unrealistic expectations—and that's not okay.

Let's face it. Certain statements in advertising are misleading, confusing, or downright impossible. I call marketing the Industry of Illusion.

Fortunately, not all cosmetics fall into this category. Many excellent moisturizers and sunscreens genuinely support healthy skin, and their marketing usually tells the consumer the plain truth about what they do.

> *"Many excellent moisturizers and sunscreens genuinely support healthy skin."*

Other products might also support healthy skin, but their marketing campaigns overpromise, overpackage, and overprice.* "In a 2010 article for the *Journal of Consumer Research*, Debra Trampe, Diederik A. Stapel, and Frans W. Siero wrote, 'One of the signature strengths of the advertising industry lies in its ability to transform seemingly mundane objects into highly desirable products.'"** These products make up fantasy stories that no cosmetic cream can scientifically (or legally) fulfill.

Eucerin® lotion, made by Beiersdorf, is an example of an excellent moisturizer. An ad for Eucerin® Advanced Repair Lotion says the lotion offers a solution to skin dryness for healthier looking skin. This ad doesn't overpromise, and the lotion truly does what it says it does. My personal research proved the value of this product time and again. (More on that in Chapter 10 on page 142.)

On the other hand, another product, which will remain nameless, promises to polish your skin. I know you can polish a car, shoes, and fingernails, but this is the first time—in my thirty-plus years of dermatology practice—I ever heard skin can be polished.

The ad goes on to say that the cream exfoliates and nourishes the skin. Exfoliation is unnecessary and nourishing is impossible. Polishing, exfoliation, and nourishing sound enticing, but none

---

*   Ketchum, "The Persuasion Technique of Beauty Product Advertising."

**   Ibid.

of these promises have any real meaning when it comes to supporting healthy skin.

Some might ask whether the product does exfoliate the skin. Since no scientific evidence proves that exfoliation actually supports skin health, I won't pursue that topic in this discussion. My clear purpose is to be your skin's advocate and focus on the issue of supporting healthy skin. That means staying off the hundreds of side trails that come up along the way.

"My goal is to help women make informed choices, whatever those choices might be."

Some women love the way their skin feels after using body polish. They aren't worried about its moisturizing qualities. In that case, they are making a choice based on what they like. I have no problem with that. My goal is to help women make informed choices, whatever those choices might be.

What started out in college as curiosity to understand those scientific names on cosmetic labels turned into my constant quest for truth. I wanted to guide my patients toward products that truly help them. So, I brought a Corneometer®* into my office. Used in clinical trials to study surface skin hydration, reputable manufacturers use this machine to be sure their products really

"What started out in college as curiosity to understand those scientific names on cosmetic labels turned into my constant quest for truth."

---

* A device that measures the hydration of the very top surface of the skin.

increase the water content of skin. NASA used a Corneometer®
on the ISS space station for the Skin-9 project.*

Over the past eight-plus years, I measured the hydration level
of volunteers' skin surface before and after applying moisturizer
and compiled the results. I asked patients to use a product on one
side of their body and a different product on the other side for
comparison. My personal findings appear in Chapter 10 on page
137, but I want to emphasize here that quality, effective skincare
products are available. Several reputable companies make effective moisturizers that truly increase the water content of skin. I
speak with confidence because I personally did the research.

Science confirms that well-formulated moisturizers and
sunscreen are two product types that truly support healthy
skin. Quality moisturizers increase skin hydration to keep skin
healthy. Applying sunscreen prevents signs of aging and helps
prevent skin cancer.** I always say, "The best wrinkle cream is a
good sunscreen."

Although moisturizers and sunscreen aren't sexy, they are the
bread and butter of maintaining healthy skin.

> *"Moisturizers and sunscreen are the bread and butter of
> maintaining healthy skin."*

Charming images and sensuous promises are very appealing—with gorgeous ads that promise your wrinkles will disap-
pear, your age spots will fade, your skin will look younger . . .
and so will you. Those messages capture the attention and the
imagination of women who yearn to look their absolute best.

---

*   Henrich, "Experiment Record N° 9392: Skin B."
** Halpern, "The Melanoma Letter," 2012 Vol 30 no. 2.

Many ads pull a one-two punch starting with common concerns about physical appearance—for example, dry scaly skin. First, they magnify the concern. They might show a woman afraid to go to a party because of her dry skin. Then, they portray someone using their product, who suddenly has a wonderful social life. Off to the party she goes, with an image of her dancing with a partner by the end of the commercial.

Marketing companies go so far as to conduct focus groups and surveys to find the most common insecurities in women, and then emphasize those topics in their ads to make women feel more and more dissatisfied with themselves.* They focus on pain because "people only take action when the pain of inaction overcomes our natural desire to conserve energy (inertia)."** In other words, you only buy when you feel bad enough about yourself.

Is your hair too straight? Put this on to curl it. If it's too curly, use this product to straighten it. Too little hair? Here's something to grow it. And if they have too much hair, here's a cream to get rid of it. Their message: you are not good enough the way you are.

Although this industry makes wonderful products that truly support healthy skin, unfortunately they also use marketing tactics that:

- Make seductive-but-unproven claims.
- Imply you need extra products that don't actually help the skin.
- Withhold vital information from the consumer.
- Redefine beauty as eternal youth.
- Use fear to increase sales.

---

* FECYT, "Do we buy cosmetics because they are useful or because they make us feel good?"

** Davret, "How To Create Pain And Sell More."

- Pull at heartstrings to get people to buy.
- Play word games that confuse the consumer.
- Create and propagate myths and more myths.
- Make you feel inadequate.

Add packaging shenanigans to all of the above and who wouldn't be confused and overwhelmed? Oddly shaped dispensers in varying sizes and different price points, bold colors, and cryptic wording—who has time to sift through it all and find a good choice?

Fortunately, you can still make good choices once you understand some basic marketing methods. Here are some of them.

Seductive Claims

Skincare aisles overflow with facial products labeled with terms like *anti-aging*, *age-defying*, and *age defense*. Although these facial moisturizers might have the benefits of hydration, they don't actually intend to change the skin. Otherwise, the law would classify them as drugs.

FryFace Rule #1
Science has yet to discover a single product or ingredient that can reverse the aging process.

Commercials for these products often show a celebrity endorser who looks fantastic for her age, acting as an illustration of what the product can do for the woman watching at home. This celebrity spent hours, even days, of preparation for the photo shoot, working with an entire team including estheticians, hair stylists, and makeup professionals. Then, she's photographed from her best angles with optimized lighting and filters and, finally, photoshopped. Sure, she looks fantastic. Who wouldn't after all that?

Most of us wipe the mist from the mirror after a shower and peer into a very different image. Why? Because it's real. Marketing is an industry of illusion. That image in the mirror is the one to embrace. She's fabulous just the way she is—the caring you, the playful you, the sexy you, the you that faces the world every single day to make a difference. Why would you want to change that woman in the mirror when she's already so amazing? Why? Because messages that she's not enough* bombard her eyes and ears up to ten thousand per day.**

Seductive claims set women up for frustration and discouragement. The *Journal of Consumer Research* reported that the simple act of looking at ads for beauty-enhancing products often makes consumers feel worse about themselves.*** I see the same frustration and discouragement on the faces of wonderful women every single day in my office. I wish I had the right words to make them understand, "You are awesome just like you are," so they would believe it and embrace it—because it is the truth.

> *"Seductive claims set women up for frustration and discouragement."*

Products You Don't Need

A skincare regimen for women with healthy skin is actually pretty simple: wash, moisturize, and apply sunscreen. Complicated skincare regimens are nothing but marketing tools to encourage the sale of more products, and they often come in cute little kits

---

*   Ketchum, "The Persuasion Technique of Beauty Product Advertising."

**   Simpson, "Finding Brand Success In the Digital World."

***   Ibid.

for you. Here's an example of a routine that gained momentum recently. (Seriously, you can't make this stuff up!)

10-Step Morning Skincare Regimen

Monday morning begins with:

STEP 1. Oil-based Cleanse

Use oil to remove makeup and "impurities" (whatever those are). Recommended oils for this step include macadamia oil, jojoba oil, or any other oil you might have in your kitchen cabinet. After wiping your face with oil, rinse with water.

STEP 2. Water-based Cleanse

Now apply a second cleanser to remove the impurities left behind by the first cleanser because it didn't finish the job. This is to remove water-soluble dirt that the previous water rinse didn't remove and to eliminate the stubborn sweat that refused to let go during the first cleanse. Recommended product: green tea.

STEP 3. Exfoliator

Now that your face is sterile, it's time to strip away the superficial layers of skin. According to the "skin experts," an exfoliator also cleans the pores.

STEP 4. Toner

Toner is the ultimate product to remove any residue left behind after the oil-based cleanser, the water-based cleanser, the mechanical polishing, and the pore drilling that went on in the previous steps. Recommended product for this step: licorice (black, not red).

STEP 5. Essence

An essence, whatever that is, supposedly hydrates, helps restore skin cells, and is anti-aging. Essence* covers a variety of ingredients from snail slime to bee propolis.

---

* Bennett, "The best Korean essences to add to your skincare routine."

STEP 6. Treatments

Now we get down to business. This is where we apply those little ampoules of powerhouse ingredients to get rid of all those lines, wrinkles, pigmented spots, and red blood vessels. This is the step that makes you look like Marilyn Monroe or Princess Diana. It's all done with vitamin C or soybeans! By now, it's Tuesday.

STEP 7. Sheet Mask

Here's where you take some arbitrary substance, maybe a cucumber or a rose, and apply it to your facial skin and let it sit there for a really long time. If you weren't late for work before, you will be now. This step is supposed to relax you, though personally, I'd be in a panic trying to get out the door. The "skin experts" also say your skin absorbs all those essential nutrients from, you know, any substance you choose to use.

STEP 8. Eye Cream

These miracle creams claim to remove dark circles, puffiness, crow's feet, and stains off of your teeth (Okay, I made the last one up). You must apply this cream with your pinky or else . . . Or what? Is one finger better than the other? Not according to science.

At least this step is a quick one. The special ingredients in the eye creams that perform all this magic are honey, ginseng, or caffeine though none has any science behind it. Remember, eye cream is just a moisturizer.

STEP 9. Moisturizer

This is one you do need. Why? Because the Essence you applied hours ago and those little ampoules of magic you delicately dabbed on with your pinky, along with the sheet mask and eye cream, were clearly not moisturizing enough. Yes, science says that well-hydrated skin is beneficial but how much moisture can one face hold?

Perhaps if we skipped the first eight steps and went right to a well-formulated moisturizer you'd be on time for work. Keep in mind, by now it's Wednesday evening.

STEP 10. Sunscreen

All kidding aside, sunscreen is the true magic potion for anti-aging. Sunscreen should be applied daily, liberally, and often. If you could pick only one skincare product to use, this is the one.

Now that you finished the 10 Steps, you're completely exhausted and you missed three days of work. And for what? A well-formulated moisturizer and sunscreen with SPF 30 or above would give your skin everything it needs in five minutes or less.

> *"People who don't know me give me strange looks when I tell them a simple skincare regimen is all your skin needs."*

People who don't know me give me strange looks when I tell them a simple skincare regimen is all your skin needs. A short list of product categories that have little proven value for healthy skin are exfoliants, masks, scrubs, toners, primers, astringents, and essences, along with dozens of other "essentials" touted by media ads.

Drawing from the knowledge I gained from my medical training, chemistry studies, and thirty years in practice, my recommendation includes two products to support healthy skin—moisturizer and sunscreen. If you hear me repeat this recommendation several times per chapter, it's because I want to break through the years of conditioning and programming that keep women stuck in a cycle of buying products that don't actually help.

The next time you reach for a beauty product on a shelf or pick up your remote to hit the buy button on a TV shopping network, take some time to consider why you feel an impulse to purchase that product. Is it the slick marketing? Don't judge yourself. These campaigns use psychology, subliminal messages, and even raise the volume on commercials, so you can hear them from the kitchen or the bathroom. You're only human. But, once you realize what's happening, you can make a conscious decision about whether to buy that pretty jar or walk away.

Withholding Vital Information from the Consumer

Slick marketing leaves out important facts that consumers need in order to make informed buying decisions. For example:

- Scrubbing skin and using harsh cleansers can remove proteins and oils the skin needs.
- Someone with particularly oily skin or someone with a skin condition might need a mild cleanser. Most people can effectively wash with only water.
- Sunscreen is the only cream that studies consistently prove to prevent the signs of photoaging* that show up as pigments, fine wrinkling, and dark spots.
- Once wrinkles happen, no cream or moisturizer is proven to remove them.

Withholding information has become a common practice, so it's important to do your own research.

Repackaging

We often take for granted standard moisturizing body lotions. They are available everywhere. Most people have a pump bottle of lotion beside the sink where they wash their hands. Generally

---

* Photoaging is the change in skin tone as a result of exposure to the sun. Compare the skin tone on the arms to the skin on the buttocks and the difference is significant. This is sun damage or photoaging.

found in the Personal Care aisle, body lotion costs around $18 per pound, give or take a few dollars, depending on where you live and where you shop.

The manufacturer might repackage that same moisturizer in a bottle with a picture of a smiling baby, then market it as a moisturizing baby lotion at $40 per pound. They might also put it into a very small tube to sell as eye cream for about $500 per pound, or in a purse-size tube as an intensive hand cream at $60 per pound. These are round numbers that vary somewhat based on where you live and the brand, but you get the picture.

The ingredients are the same. The package is the only difference. By repackaging the same cream, the company can place the product in four different locations in the same store and adjust the price for the going rate in that aisle.

Here are examples of two effective moisturizers manufactured by the same company where both packages list the same ingredients.

Example 1.
- Neutrogena® Hydro Boost Hyaluronic Acid Gel Cream Moisturizer for Extra Dry Skin in a 1.7-ounce jar
- Neutrogena® Hydro Boost Hyaluronic Acid Gel Eye Cream in a 0.5-ounce tube.

Example 2.
- Aquaphor® Healing Ointment
- Aquaphor® Baby Healing Ointment

A company might go a step further by adding *anti-aging* to the label. To back up those words, they may add a miniscule amount of a particular ingredient to satisfy the anti-aging claim. This is what I call a *marketing tool ingredient*. Although no clinically significant studies prove these added substances make any impact on the skin, they are enticing to the consumer and improve sales.

For example, they might add the marketing tool ingredient CoEnzyme Q, then place the cream in a beautiful jar about the size of a shot glass to sell for $300 an ounce or $4,800 a pound. In that jar is the same moisturizer going for $18 per pound in the Personal Care aisle, only now with CoEnzyme Q.

What does CoEnzyme Q do in this case? It gives a reason to put *anti-aging* on the label. If this sounds like circular reasoning, that's because it is.

Remember, we're talking about a cosmetic that, by law, cannot intend to change the skin permanently. No ingredient exists that can turn back the clock.

When CBS came to my office, they put my chemistry knowledge to the test. They covered the product label on a small tube, so only the ingredient list showed. The producer handed me the product, then asked, "What is this?" After scanning the label, I said, "This is your typically formulated moisturizer."

She replied, "No. Actually, Dr. Frey, it's an eye cream."

To which I replied, "No, it's actually a moisturizer." That opened the door for me to teach them the majority of products such as eye creams, night creams, anti-aging creams, firming creams, and on and on are moisturizers formulated from the same basic recipe. Just because the dispenser looks different doesn't mean the contents inside are different. (I go into this in more detail in Chapter 8 on page 113.)

> *"Just because the dispenser looks different doesn't mean the contents inside are different."*

Defining Beauty as Eternal Youth

In our starstruck culture, cosmetic marketers define beauty as youthfulness. Hollywood views a young woman at the age of twenty-five as past her prime. Yet would anyone say that Sigourney Weaver or Susan Sarandon are anything less than beautiful? How about Julia Roberts, Nicole Kidman, or Sandra Bullock— all now in their fifties? Youth is not an accomplishment.

Is it true a woman has to look like a college sophomore in order to be beautiful? The very idea would be laughable if it weren't so sad. What a crushing weight these advertising campaigns put on accomplished, vibrant, amazing women. While it's true the faces of women change with age, it's merely a mindset that says this change makes them less attractive.

The cosmetic industry thrives in a perfect storm: the combination of a celebrity-obsessed culture with celebrity-endorsed products, media outlets profiting from both manufacturers and advertisers of these same products, and an aging population desperate to believe their anti-aging claims.

The term *anti-aging* is probably the most brilliant and most effective marketing term in the history of skincare. Unfortunately, the term *anti-aging* has no medical definition. According to the FDA, it is simply a marketing term.*

"Youth is not an accomplishment."

Word Games

Playing with words is a basic part of marketing. This topic fills textbooks, and the information is easily available. I listed these below because they happen so often in cosmetic marketing.

---

* FDA, "Wrinkle Treatments and Other Anti-aging Products."

32

1. Marketing Language That Uses Medical Terms

Many words printed on the front of skincare product labels have no standard definition according to the FDA. While they might have a medical meaning, they cannot be considered valid claims or promises for a product's benefits. I go into this in detail in later chapters, but to make this point as it applies to marketing, here are a few easily recognizable examples:

- Hypoallergenic: This is a medical expression, but no product test can guarantee that a consumer will not have an allergic reaction to a certain product. It is a marketing term.
- Non-comedogenic: This term implies that a product is less likely to cause breakouts. However, even when limiting your choices to non-comedogenic products, no one can guarantee the user a clear complexion. It is a marketing term.
- Nourishing: The superficial layer of skin where you apply products is made up of dead cells. It is not medically possible to nourish dead tissue. It is a marketing term.
- Dermatologist tested: No standardized guidelines exist for who the dermatologist is, their relationship to the product, or how the testing was done. It is a marketing term.

"Many words used in cosmetics marketing have no industry standard or FDA definition."

2. Rhetorical Questions

Marketers use persuasive questions to make people feel a certain way about a brand. A rhetorical question expects no answer. These questions are carefully engineered to bring up a positive response. The mind will always answer a question, so this method is a powerful way to fill a consumer's mind with assumptions that may or may not be true. "It is well known to be an effective persuasive device in advertising."*

This can work in a couple of ways. For example:

Q: What's the best scrub for healthy skin?

A: Our minds immediately begin to sort through various brands for an answer, but the correct response is: none of them. Scrubs don't support healthy skin, so no best one exists. This is definitely a trick question.

Q: Better than Botox?

A: Most people don't see the question mark. They assume this product would do what Botox can do but without the injections. Because these marketers framed their idea as a question, the concept can't be challenged by science or by the people owning Botox. The correct response: the advertised cream is a cosmetic and, by law, can't intend to change the structure or function of the skin.

Scare Tactics

Sometimes ads use scare tactics to claim that their product is better because it does not contain a dangerous ingredient. Often, these so-called dangerous ingredients are not dangerous at all.

For example: petrolatum, also known as petroleum jelly, has been villainized because it comes from the petroleum industry. Petroleum jelly is likely the safest skincare product on the market. It's so safe that clinical trials often use it as the negative control because virtually no one is allergic to it, and it has no side

---

* Pererva, "The Reasonableness of Rhetorical Questions in Advertisements."

effects even after long-term use. It's one of my favorite skincare products. However, you'll see "petrolatum-free" on some labels as though that is some sort of benefit.

Cosmetic companies are very careful to maintain high safety standards. We know this so well we take it for granted. People in the audience always smile when I say, "No one ever died from cold cream." Each year in the US, foodborne diseases sicken 48 million people, put 128,000 in the hospital, and cause 3,000 deaths.* The skincare industry has approximately four hundred reported adverse events each year.** This industry's safety record is stellar.

Scare tactics are simply a way to draw attention, and that's marketing plain and simple.

Buzzwords That Tug the Heartstrings

Labels often announce "Cruelty-Free" or "Not Tested on Animals" to make an emotional appeal to animal lovers.*** But what does that expression mean, exactly?

Some manufacturers apply this claim to only the finished product. The same manufacturers might rely on ingredient suppliers who perform animal testing. Also, the ingredients or the final product might not be currently tested on animals, but they were tested on animals in the past. With no legal definition, the manufacturer can apply its own meaning to the terms "Cruelty Free" and "Not Tested on Animals." These are marketing terms.

"Safe for the Planet" and "Green" are also heartstring phrases. In addition to nonbiodegradable ingredients like polypropylene

---

* Centers for Disease Control and Prevention, "Burden of Foodborne Illness: Findings."

** JAMA Network, "How Many Adverse Events Are Reported to FDA for Cosmetics, Personal Care?"

*** Lohrey, "Advertising Theories of Cosmetics."

beads, I'm also concerned about the amount of packaging around each little tube or jar. If a company truly wants to be safe for the planet, they would eliminate these plastics and other packaging that is not biodegradable.

Bizarre Discoveries

Every few months, a new discovery comes out in the ads. The most bizarre materials are announced as new and marvelous breakthroughs, from snail slime to nightingale poop.* As crazy as it sounds, celebrities often encourage and market these trends. Marketers might call these breakthrough products, but with no science as backup, these crazes are examples of sensational fads at best.**

When a group of people accept a belief and pass those ideas on, those ideas become social myths. Some of the myths I heard growing up were: Don't cross your eyes or they'll get stuck like that. If you go outside with wet hair, you'll get a cold. Pull out a grey hair and two more will appear in its place. Crack your knuckles and you will end up with arthritis. An apple a day keeps the doctor away, and Twinkies *don't* have an expiration date.

The same is true in skincare. Some well-known myths include:

- Chemical-free skincare products are better.
- Stem cell creams rejuvenate the skin.
- You must drink eight glasses of water a day for healthy skin.
- Face cleanser prevents wrinkles.
- Shaving makes hair grow back thicker.

---

* Mae, ". . . The Nightingale Poop Anti Aging Facial."

** Dictionary.com, "Fad: a temporary fashion, notion, manner of conduct, etc., especially one followed enthusiastically by a group."

- "Natural" products are safer.
- Women over fifty should use products for mature skin.

When it comes down to it, this multi-billion-dollar industry that produces so many quality products, also has one dominating message: Women aren't good enough like they are. In order to look their best, women must invest a lot of time and spend a lot of money.

That's the bottom line, isn't it?

CHAPTER 3

Cultural Practices without Scientific Basis

U p until now, we've been talking about marketing messages that confuse the consumer. These shenanigans don't stop with word games. Marketing companies also take advantage of cultural norms with no scientific basis. Here are some universal myths related to face washing:

- Scrub your face every morning, so your skin looks fresh and glowing. (What exactly defines a glowing face? Is shiny bad and glowing good? Why or why not?)
- You should wash your face before bed, or you'll get break-outs. (Maybe. But maybe not.)

- Wash your face before bed, or you'll get wrinkles.
- Going to bed with makeup on will cause both breakouts and wrinkles.

While a scientific study supports face washing twice daily for adolescent acne,* none of the above statements have any scientific basis for those with healthy skin. Still, entire product lines related to washing have become a cultural norm. Some people experience healthier skin by eliminating products altogether and using plain water instead.** The truth is, maintaining healthy skin can be very simple and affordable.

"Maintaining healthy skin can be very simple and affordable."

Women's magazines routinely publish articles explaining which products to use and why. They write reviews on which ones are best—when some of those products are optional and many aren't necessary at all. Here are some of them:

Cleansers

Yes, cleansers. You are probably cringing right about now as the concept that you don't need a facial cleanser goes against what your mother taught you. Let me clarify.

First of all, as a physician, I want to emphasize that the practice of handwashing has probably made more impact on world health than any single drug or other practice. An abundance of scientific evidence shows that handwashing minimizes

---

* Choi, "A single-blinded, randomized, controlled clinical trial evaluating the effect of face washing on acne vulgaris."

** Vartan, "Are You Washing Your Face Too Much?"

digestive-tract illnesses and pneumonias, as well as decreasing the spread of viral illness such as the common cold.

The World Health Organization (WHO) includes hand-washing as part of their infection control practices. The Centers for Disease Control and Prevention (CDC) recommends we wash our hands during and after food preparation, before eating, when caring for the ill, before and after treating a wound, after using the toilet or a diaper change, after blowing your nose, coughing or sneezing, after touching animals or their waste, and after touching garbage.* Handwashing with a cleanser is important.

> *"Handwashing is important."*

Daily showering or bathing is a far different matter.

The skin's primary role is to provide a protective barrier. Along with the physical barrier, the surface of normal healthy skin has a population of beneficial microorganisms—known as the skin's microbiome. These organisms support our immune system and keep harmful pathogens from entering the body.

Cleansers make no distinction between harmful or beneficial microorganisms. Daily showering and bathing remove many beneficial microorganisms and weaken our first line of defense against pathogens. This allows hardier pathogens to grow, some-times to the point of becoming resistant to antibiotics. Staying away from cleansers, especially harsh cleansers, might be better when it comes to skin health.

> *"Cleansers make no distinction between harmful or beneficial microorganisms."*

---

* CDC, "Keeping Hands Clean."

When I speak on this topic, people often give me a doubt-ful stare when I say, "Showering has few health benefits." Even among board-certified dermatologists there is no consensus regarding how often a person with healthy skin needs to cleanse. No one can say for sure how often we should shower or bathe or if using a cleanser will improve your health.

Even without a cleanser, frequent hot showers can strip away healthy lipids and proteins the skin uses to maintain adequate hydration. Dry, flaky skin is less effective than healthy skin at preventing infection from dangerous microbes.

> *"Frequent hot showers can strip the skin of healthy lipids and proteins."*

The result of harsh cleansers and over-washing:

- An impaired skin barrier.
- Dry, flaky skin.
- Antibiotic-resistant pathogens.
- The perfect storm for infection and skin reactions.

Studies show that showering habits differ from culture to culture.* In the US, India, Mexico, and Spain, the average is one shower per day. In Brazil, the average is eleven showers per week. In the Himba tribe of Namibia, Africa, the average is never. Bathing with water is not part of their culture.**

---

* Euromonitor Research, "Survey Shows Regional Differences in Bathing Habits Around the World."

** Ademola, "The real reason why the Himba people in Namibia don't bathe."

A shower removes irritating chemicals after swimming in a pool. A shower removes irritating salt after swimming a romp in the ocean. Workers exposed to harmful chemicals might benefit from after-work showers. For most people, that's not the case.

People shower for many reasons: because they like it, to wake up, to wash off workout sweat, to prevent body odor, or because someone taught them that showering is what nice people do.

If an individual prefers to shower daily, I'd recommend:

- Brief, lukewarm showers.
- The use of a mild soap-free cleanser, for those who prefer a cleanser.
- Applying a well-formulated moisturizer after toweling dry.

Face Washing

Have you ever considered how much dirt adheres to a woman's face in the course of a day? Unless she's working in a coal mine or paving roads, probably not very much. Marketing jargon often mentions removing pollution from our faces. Has anyone ever identified what facial pollution is exactly? If this is really an issue, shouldn't we be advising city folks to wash their faces more than country folks? Does any of this make sense?

If you believe the commercials, a clean face is difficult to achieve and requires at least three products, if not more. Science does not back this up. No studies exist proving the need for a cleanser for washing the face.

Dermatological literature has no definitive recommendation as to how often to wash your face or what products to use. Research shows no real consensus for mature women with healthy skin.*

---

* Adolescents with acne should wash twice a day using a mild cleanser.

Several years ago, I surveyed five hundred female patients between the ages of thirty-five and seventy years of age, none with any inflammatory skin conditions. Fifty percent washed their faces only using warm water. These women had beautiful healthy skin, and their cleansing routine took a couple of minutes during their morning shower. (By the way, personally, I don't use face cleanser as part of my daily routine.)

> *"Fifty percent of my female patients use only water to wash their faces."*

How Cleansers Work

Cleansing products contain ingredients called surfactants which surround and lift dirt, sebum, loose skin cells, makeup, and pollution, if any are present, so water can wash them away. Surfactants can't distinguish between wanted substances like proteins and lipids from unwanted substances such as oils and dirt. When using a cleanser, you're literally throwing the baby out with the bath water. While a cleanser might remove particles from your face, it can also leave your skin feeling dry and irritated.

Friction or rubbing might also help remove dirt from the skin. We naturally rub our hands over the area while washing. Some people prefer to use a washcloth on the face, but is that washcloth clean? Does it contain unwanted bacteria? How about those loofah scrubs? Are they sanitary? After hanging in a warm moist shower for days, could bacteria possibly be growing on them? I recommend washing with your hands instead of using a washcloth.

> *"I recommend washing with your hands instead of using a washcloth."*

Besides the question of staying sanitary, is all that scrubbing, buffing, and abrading of the skin really necessary? Credible studies showing health benefits from scouring the skin are nonexistent. However, plenty of studies and anecdotal evidence prove too much rubbing can cause skin irritation. I can only imagine what it does to the microbiome.

Soap

Most people think the words *soap* and *cleanser* are synonymous. They are not. A true soap is a combination of a strong alkali and fat from animal, vegetable, or mineral sources. Lye (sodium hydroxide or potassium hydroxide) is traditionally the alkali ingredient.

Pioneer women melted animal fat, then mixed in wood ashes which contained lye. They boiled that combination in big pots out in the yard until the thick mass was ready to pour out to cool and cut it into bars. They used those bars for everything from scrubbing floors to washing clothes, to bathing and shampooing.

> *"A true soap is a combination of fat and a strong alkali."*

True soaps have a very high pH of 9–10 and can be harsh on your skin. While soap removes dirt, sebum, and makeup, it also strips away lipids and proteins your skin needs to stay healthy. True soaps can dry and irritate the skin, especially for those with certain conditions such as eczema.* Very few true soaps are available on the market today. The Original Ivory® bar is a true soap.

Manufacturers wanted a product that was less irritating and less drying than true soap, so they developed synthetic detergent

---

* FDA, "Frequently Asked Questions on Soap."

bars, or syndet bars. Like soap, synthetic surfactants also surround and lift dirt and oils, so water can wash them away. They don't clean as well as true soaps, but they also don't strip away the skin's beneficial and necessary proteins and lipids as readily either. With a more favorable pH in the 5–7 range, this type of cleanser contains less than 10 percent true soap. Dove® and Oil of Olay® are examples of syndet bars.

> *"Syndet bars are less irritating and drying than true soap."*

For those who want more cleaning action, combo bars are combination cleansers that combine soap and syndets to create a product that's more effective than syndet bars and easier on the skin than true soap. Many of these add fragrance, such as Dial® and Irish Spring®.

> *"Comb cleansers are more effective and easier on the skin."*

Soap-Free Cleansers

Because they are less drying, I recommend soap-free cleansers to my patients who want to use a cleanser. Here are several types:

- Oil-free cleansers contain no fats. Many contain glycerin and sodium lauryl sulfate. They don't clean as well as soaps, but they also aren't as irritating. These cleansers are ideal for people with dry skin in areas that don't need excessive cleansing. Cetaphil® Gentle Skin Cleanser* is an example.

---

* https://www.amazon.com/Cetaphil-Gentle-Cleanser-Types-Ounce/dp/B07GC74LL5/ref=sr_1_4

- Cleansing creams, like the famous Pond's® Cold Cream Cleanser,* contain occlusives, such as petrolatum, beeswax, or mineral oil. These creams are ideal for removing oil-based foundation, makeup, and dirt while also moisturizing.
- Oil cleansers are the latest craze, based on the concept that oil dissolves oil. They contain no surfactants. These products use many different types of oils from mineral oil to argan oil to jojoba oil and others. I rarely recommend oil cleansers, as some people with normal healthy skin might experience breakouts from them. Acne patients beware!
- Micellar water is very in-vogue at this writing. This product is mostly water with a very small concentration of surfactant. When micellar water is applied to skin, the surfactants surround the unwanted oil and form tiny clusters called micelles. These micelles lift the unwanted elements from the skin, so water can easily wash them away. The profitability of these products is massive since their main ingredient is water. Micellar water is simply a soap-free water-based cleanser that might be useful to remove eye makeup. It can be ideal for women with sensitive skin.

"I recommend soap-free cleansers to my patients who want to use a cleanser."

So, which is best? Cleansers run the full span from harsh soaps to very mild micellar water. Again, this depends on the

---

* https://www.amazon.com/Ponds-Cold-Cream-Cleanser-3-5/dp/ B000052YQN/ref=sr_1_4

individual's wants and needs. Remember, about 50 percent of my female patients with normal healthy skin don't use any cleanser at all. I don't either. Check the ingredient listing and see what works best for you.

Makeup Removers

No specific ingredients define a makeup remover. Water removes makeup. Milk also removes makeup—whole milk, skim milk, or chocolate milk. (Joke.) Take your pick.

On skincare aisles, you'll find liquid makeup removers, micellar water removers, and cleansing wipes in both wet and dry versions, along with toner makeup removers and natural oil removers like jojoba, coconut, and argan oils. Corn oil, canola oil, and baby oil would work just as well at a lower price point.* You'll find makeup removers for specific areas of the face, like eye-makeup removers and lip-makeup removers on this aisle, too.

A makeup remover is any formulation marketed to remove makeup. Basically, it's a cleanser. Unless you wear heavy oil-based makeup, plain water will likely do the job.

Now for the million-dollar question: Does a woman with healthy skin really need to remove her makeup before she goes to bed? Her face was comfortable wearing that makeup all day long. Are we supposed to believe that lying down with the lights off in a quiet house transforms that same makeup into some kind of menace? No valid science shows that leaving makeup on at night causes wrinkles, premature aging, or breakouts.

Some recommend removing makeup because skin needs to breathe at night. Lungs breathe. Skin does not breathe.

"No science shows that leaving makeup on at night causes wrinkles, premature aging, or breakouts."

---

* Acne sufferers beware of using oils!

If you like to keep your pillowcase clean, rinse your face with water before bed. If you prefer, use a mild cleanser, then rinse with water. Your laundry basket will thank you, but your face probably doesn't care either way.

Shampoo

Ask your mother or grandmother what shampoo she used as a child, and she'll probably tell you she can't remember. Shampoo, as we know it today, didn't appear on store shelves until the late 1950s. Bottled shampoo became a household staple thanks to Mr. Breck who popularized the Breck girls through TV commercials. Prior to that, most people used bar soap to wash their hair, which was the traditional soap made from animal fat and lye. Bar soap often left soap scum, an off-white unpleasant residue, on the hair because many homes used hard water from the family well.

Manufacturers of Breck®, Prell®, and Johnson & Johnson® Baby Shampoo had an eager public wanting a product that left their hair feeling soft, smooth, and manageable after washing. Now, seventy years later, the use of shampoo is deeply embedded in the global culture.

"Shampoo is deeply embedded in the global culture."

Recently, no-poo campaigns have begun questioning the need for shampoo. These no-poo enthusiasts have a point, as science shows no evidence that using shampoo provides health benefits. Although modern shampoos make it easier to get pleasing cosmetic outcomes—as in clean, silky, manageable hair—science has shown that too much shampooing can also damage the hair.*

Shampoos are formulated with three main types of ingredients:

---

* Zhang, "Effect of shampoo, conditioner, and permanent waving on the molecular structure of human hair."

1. Functional ingredients that make the shampoo work. These include:

- Surfactants—surround and lift dirt and oils so water can wash them away.
- Sequestering agents—prevent soap scum from forming on the hair and scalp.
- Preservatives—necessary for all water-based products to prevent growth of bacteria and fungus.

2. Aesthetic ingredients, so the consumer likes the look and feel of the shampoo itself.

Most people won't buy a shampoo that pours out of the bottle like clear water with no color. Thickeners give the shampoo substance. Other ingredients make the product opaque, colored, and even sparkly, so the shampoo looks pretty in the palm of your hand. These ingredients don't improve the shampoo's cleansing ability, but they do improve sales.

Foaming agents have no cleansing value, but consumers like lather. Fragrance also has no cleansing value, but it is probably the most important aspect of a shampoo's attraction.

Much of a shampoo's ingredient list has nothing to do with effectiveness and more to do with creating a pleasant user experience, since a desirable user experience increases sales.

"Much of a shampoo's ingredient list has nothing to do with effectiveness and more to do with creating a pleasant user experience."

3. Marketing ingredients

Although they don't necessarily add any scientifically proven benefits, marketing ingredients appease the claims on the shampoo label. For example, adding vitamin C to shampoo supposedly protects the hair from the damaging effects of the sun's ultraviolet rays. Unfortunately, little science proves this claim. As a water-soluble compound, vitamin C washes down the drain when you rinse.

One caveat regarding the instructions on many shampoo bottles: I don't follow them. I just wash and rinse. No need to repeat.

> *"I just wash and rinse. No need to repeat."*

Masks

Egyptians used donkey milk, honey, and clay to draw out impurities. In the eighteenth century, the English mixed mashed-up strawberries and raw veal to revitalize their skin. Ubtan masks in India were made of turmeric, often mixed with coconut oil and aloe vera to clarify the skin. Imperial China combined pearls, lotus root, ground ginger, and crushed tea leaves to purify the skin. Ancient Rome relied on starch and eggs, placenta, and excrements from calves to preserve the complexion.*

Some things have not changed.

Nightingale poop, anyone?

Even today, masks are seemingly arbitrary products applied to the skin and left on for an arbitrary amount of time, often with skincare claims that overpromise. These claims say masks:

- Provide deep moisturization—compared to superficial moisturization? And how does one measure this?
- Replenish the skin—with what? With water? If the label infers that the mask helps hydration, a well-formulated moisturizer will do the same.

---

* Nandi, "The Fascinating History of Face Masks from Around the World."

- Remove the sebum or oil—how about splashing a little water on your face? That'll work. Or use a mild cleanser if you want.
- Remove skin debris—what is debris exactly? I hear people say, "You have ketchup on your chin," but I never hear anyone say, "You have debris on your face."
- Detoxify—in medical school we learn the word *detoxify* applies to ridding the body of illicit drugs. It has nothing to do with the skin. Besides, which toxins accumulate in the skin? I can't name one.
- Rejuvenate the skin—miraculously, the skin rejuvenates on its own. About one layer of outer skin sheds off each day. The thin top layer of the epidermis, called the stratum corneum, replaces itself every sixteen days* all by itself. The entire epidermis replaces itself every twenty-eight days. Again, all by itself.
- Rest the skin—I recently saw an ad that said a sheet mask allows the skin to rest. How can you tell if your skin is tired? Did it overwork today? In my thirty years as a dermatologist, I never read any science that says skin cells take rest breaks or go on vacation. The stratum corneum is made up of dead cells, so they are already resting in peace.
- Refresh . . .
- Revitalize . . .
- Tone . . .
- Reduce wrinkles . . .
- Washes your windows . . . just kidding.

---

* Iizuka, "Epidermal Turnover Time."

The truth is, science doesn't prove any of these claims to be true or that masks are more effective than a well-formulated moisturizer.

Another problem with masks is their lack of standardized methods. Exactly how long does a mask stay on? Three minutes, five minutes, twenty minutes, a week? Who makes that decision?

> *"Another problem with masks is their lack of standardized methods."*

These arbitrary application times are just that, arbitrary. Unfortunately, some of these products can be harmful when left on too long. They can cause irritation, rashes, and also sensitize the skin. Masks can also remove lipids and proteins necessary for skin hydration. Peel-off masks tug at the skin when you remove them, which is not ideal.

Masks might feel great and be part of a fun afternoon activity. They are also a profitable spa procedure. However, don't expect a mask to deliver on any of its promises. Also, be careful. Harmful side effects like acne breakouts or an itchy inflamed rash called contact dermatitis from mask application are not a rare occurrence.[*]

> *"Harmful side effects from mask application are not a rare occurrence."*

---

[*] Khanna, "Rejuvenating Facial Massage--A Bane or Boon?"

Facials

A facial is a multistep process for your face. This process usually includes a consultation, cleansing, exfoliation, extraction, steam, application of a variety of masks, potions, and products, as well as a relaxing massage. The person who administers the facial can range from an untrained high school graduate to a professional licensed aesthetician.

Marketing claims for facials are similar to those for masks. They promise to cleanse the pores and remove dead skin cells, as well as to rejuvenate, nourish, and hydrate your skin. Like masks, facials have no standard definition and little science substantiates their marketing claims.

Facials can be relaxing and fun. They can also be dangerous. About one-third of people who participate in a facial will experience redness, swelling, delayed skin reactions, and acne-like breakouts.* Similar to many other aspects of cosmetic skincare, a facial might make a woman feel good, but whether it supports healthy skin remains in question.

> *"A facial might make a woman feel good, but whether it supports healthy skin remains in question."*

If you want to have a party with your friends and have fun smearing arbitrary stuff on your face—go ahead—just don't expect the process to improve your facial skin health.

Here is my recommendation for a cleansing routine:

In the morning, wash your face with water in the shower. If you choose to use a cleanser, use something mild. In the evening, if you choose to wash your face, simply use water. If you use heavy or oil-based makeup, you might want to use a mild cleanser, especially if you don't like doing laundry.

---

* Ibid.

CHAPTER 4

Skin Regimen "Essentials" That Aren't Necessary

So much marketing has one underlying message: You're not good enough as you are. Well, you are! These ads imply that something about you needs fixing, and they have a product to fix it, whether the problem is real or not. This message is especially strong when it comes to unnecessary products.

The word *polishing* definitely falls within this category. You tell me. Does a woman's face need to be polished like a coffee table or a car? Do people who never polish their skin have less healthy skin than those who do? How essential is this process, anyway?

Food, water, and sunscreen are essential, which means your well-being depends on them. Polishing? Not so much.

Consumers who want to make informed decisions need to understand the differences between essential, optional, and unnecessary skincare products.

- Essential—vital for healthy skin, and everyone should use it.
- Optional—makes the skin feel good with little risk to using it, but it doesn't necessarily improve your skin's well-being.
- Unnecessary—has no proven benefit for skin health and might even cause problems.

Marketing gurus and cosmetic-counter salespeople have a long list of products they say are essential: cleansers, exfoliants, scrubs, polishing cleansers, toners, astringents, primers, night creams, essences, and serums. In other words, many of those little bottles and jars on your bathroom counter.

While these items might make your skin feel good, are any of them vitally important to facial skin health? Are they even a good idea?

Promoting healthy skin means supporting the skin's primary function as a protective barrier that keeps water in and germs out. Let's see how the following products achieve this goal.

Exfoliants, Scrubs & Polishing Cleansers

No one has proven that removing loose skin cells, also called exfoliation, is beneficial for skin health. Skin naturally falls away in its normal shedding process. Protein bridges hold together the outermost layers of skin cells. When a cell is old and ready to shed, enzymes dissolve the bridges, and the cell falls away. These enzymes need a well-hydrated environment. In a dry environment, the enzymes cannot dissolve the bridges. As a result, the cells hang on and make the skin look flaky.

"Skin naturally falls away in its normal shedding process."

The use of quality moisturizers increases the water content of skin and supports this enzyme action. When old skin cells fall away, the skin looks soft and smooth. When you keep your skin hydrated, exfoliation happens gently. While scrubbing might make your skin feel smoother, removing too many skin cells can result in irritated, dry, and even inflamed skin.

Instructions on how to use exfoliants, scrubs, and polishes vary from product to product. Some recommend using them once a week, some twice a week, and others once a month. If these arbitrary directions aren't enough to put exfoliants and scrubs in question, I've found even more reasons to doubt the need for these products.

A frequent claim on these products says that removing the top surface layers of skin boosts skin cell turnover, as though taking away the old replenishes the new faster. How do these companies measure skin cell turnover to validate this claim?

Measuring skin cell turnover is a difficult scientific endeavor even by the best of laboratory scientists. It involves radiolabeled isotopes at the cellular level or 3D imaging techniques. Both are imperfect and subjective.*

If a company did invest the massive amount of funding to use this equipment, they still couldn't account for the fact that different users have varying rates of cell turnover based on age, level of health, and other factors. For cost-conscious manufacturers, results from this expensive testing have little practical meaning. Skin cell turnover is a marketing claim without proven scientific foundation.

---

* Maeda, "New Method of Measurement of Epidermal Turnover in Humans."

"Skin cell turnover is a marketing claim without proven scientific foundation."

For certain skin ailments, under the control and guidance of a dermatologist, some patients might benefit from skin exfoliation. However, this is certainly not the same as recommending that people with healthy skin use scrubs, no matter how often.

Too much scrubbing can be drying at the least and damaging at the worst. Why not be kinder to your face and apply a high-quality moisturizer that increases skin hydration? Support your skin while gently promoting the release of skin cells that are ready to let go.

If you have healthy skin, exfoliants, scrubs, and polishes fall under the unnecessary category.

Toners & Astringents

Beauty magazines and cosmetic-counter salespeople tell us to use a toner after a cleanser. Toners come in many different formulations along with a list of alleged benefits. Like so many cosmetic skincare products, no standard ingredient formulation or definition describes a toner.

Marketing claims for toners include the following:

- Cleanse. (How much dirt can be left after you've just washed your face?)
- Remove residue from cleanser. (If you need a toner to remove residue from your cleanser, you're using the wrong cleanser.)
- Shrink pores. (Like the length of your arm, pore size does not change.)
- Remove dust, pollen, and pollution. (You just washed your face. Did you miss some spots?)

- Hydrate. (Moisturizers, not toners, increase the water content of the skin.)
- Soothe and calm. (What does this mean exactly? Does the skin have anxiety?)
- Repair. (What exactly is repaired by the toner? Skin repair happens naturally.)
- Nourish. (Remember this one from Chapter 1 on page 9? The skin is not the digestive system. Skin cells are dead, so they can't be nourished.)
- Stimulate blood circulation.
- Balance the skin's pH.
- Function as an antibacterial.
- Clear blemishes.
- And yada, yada, yada . . .

Some toners are used with water, some without. Many contain alcohol, some don't. Those that claim to "refresh" are often called tonics, not to be confused with a carbonated beverage containing quinine.

"Stronger" toners with up to 60 percent alcohol are called astringents. Astringents are drying agents that might cause redness, irritation, or burning to some individuals. Basically, astringents dry out the skin, so you need more moisturizer. Does this make sense to anyone?

Toners and astringents can be sprayed on, dabbed on, applied with gauze, a washcloth, or your fingers. Some should be rinsed off with water, while others are left on.

My advice: If you want to cleanse your skin, use plain warm water with or without a mild soap-free cleanser. Afterward, apply a well-formulated moisturizer.

Skip the toner. It's unnecessary.

Primers

Introduced into the skincare market about a decade ago, primers were initially marketed as a product that keeps makeup on the face for hours. What ingredients in primers help create this long-lasting effect? Curious, I looked at ingredients lists on many primers and couldn't find a single one. I did find that the ingredients in most primers are the same ingredients found in facial moisturizers.

> *"Ingredients in most primers are the same ingredients found in facial moisturizers."*

No published studies verify that makeup lasts longer with primer. How would anyone determine that anyway?

Ads for primers say that these products add radiance, diminish fine lines, and color-correct, although I'm not sure if they intend to color-correct the skin or the makeup. They also claim to erase pores, which sounds suspiciously similar to the claims for toner. Unfortunately, no scientific basis supports any of these assertions.

Does your facial skin need preparation for foundation and makeup? Here's another example of the underlying message: you're not good enough like you are. You need to make your natural state better.

Your face is not a wall that you need to prepare for paint. Primers are unnecessary.

Night Cream

I get a lot of smile mileage from the topic of night creams during my speaking engagements when I ask:

"Does your night cream go to work at sundown, at 10 p.m. or at midnight?"

"Is your night cream thrown off by daylight savings time?"

"Does night cream work by the time zone where it was made or the time zone where you live?"

"If you work the night shift, should you wear day cream or night cream?"

I try to use humor to inform people about skincare. I find it helpful when we can laugh at ourselves because we're all in the same boat when it comes to marketing influence.

The fact is, skin doesn't change from day to night, and ingredients can't tell time. The entire night-cream topic is beyond logic and has one sole purpose: to sell two bottles or jars instead of one. The only true difference between night cream and day cream is that night cream doesn't contain sunscreen. One might feel thicker than the other, but both of them are simply moisturizers.

Eye Cream

Eye cream is a moisturizer in a tiny tube at a higher price. Yes, the skin around the eyes is thin, but under a microscope a pathologist cannot distinguish a skin sample from the cheekbone from skin taken around the eye. Some might say that the thinnest eyelid skin is more susceptible to damage from the sun's ultraviolet rays, but ironically, most eye creams don't contain sunscreen.

With the high safety standards of reputable skincare manufacturers, facial moisturizers must be as safe near the eyes as on the cheekbone or the forehead. If a facial moisturizer isn't safe enough to apply around the eye, it certainly shouldn't be applied high on the cheekbone, less than an inch from the eye.

"Facial moisturizers must be safe near the eyes."

With more than thirty years of experience comparing ingredients listings, I've discovered many products with the same ingredients, packaged differently, and sold at varying price points.

As an example, I chose a product I regularly recommend to my patients. This product always performs well in my corneometer testing, and my test subjects like its feel.

Visiting Neutrogena.com, I found Neutrogena® Hydro Boost Gel-Cream with Hyaluronic Acid for Extra-Dry Skin.* Priced at $23.99 for a 1.7-ounce jar ($225 per pound). Their eye cream is Neutrogena® Hydro Boost Hydrating Gel Eye Cream with Hyaluronic Acid.** Priced at $22.99 for a 0.5-ounce tube ($735 per pound).

Below are the ingredient listings for both products, taken from the company's website*** and from labels of these products in my office.

FryFace Rule #2
The most important information on a skincare bottle is the ingredient listing.

Before we look at the ingredients in detail, I'd like to share with you what cosmetic chemists call the 1% Line. The FDA's labeling rule states, "Ingredients present at a concentration not exceeding 1% may be listed in any order after the listing of the ingredients present at more than 1% in descending order of

---

* https://www.neutrogena.com/skin/skin-moisturizers/neutrogena-hydro-boost-water-gel-with-hyaluronic-acid-for-dry-skin/6811047.html

** https://www.neutrogena.com/skin/skin-darkcircles/neutrogena-hydro-boost-gel-cream-eye/6811049.html

*** Neutrogena.com, March 22, 2022.

predominance."* Above the 1% Line, ingredients are in order from most to least. After the 1% Line, the order can be scrambled. Here are the ingredients from the moisturizer and eye cream side by side.

Moisturizer	Eye Cream
• Water	• Water
• Dimethicone	• Dimethicone
• Glycerin	• Glycerin
• Cetearyl Olivate	• Cetearyl Olivate
• Polyacrylamide	• Polyacrylamide
• Sorbitan Olivate	• Sorbitan Olivate
• Phenoxyethanol	• Phenoxyethanol
• Dimethicone/ vinyl Dimethicone Crosspolymer	• Dimethicone/ vinyl Dimethicone Crosspolymer
• Synthetic Beeswax	• Synthetic Beeswax
• C13-14 Isoparaffin	• C13-14 Isoparaffin
• Dimethiconol	• Dimethiconol
• Dimethicone Crosspolymer	• Dimethicone Crosspolymer
• Chlorphenesin	• Chlorphenesin
• Laureth-7	• Laureth-7
• Carbomer	• Carbomer
• Sodium Hyaluronate	• Sodium Hyaluronate
• Ethylhexylglycerin	• Ethylhexylglycerin
• C12-14 pareth-12	• C12-14 pareth-12
• Sodium Hydroxide	• Sodium Hydroxide

Finding the 1% Line in these ingredients takes a bit of formulation knowledge and sometimes some research. CosmeticsInfo.org is

---

* FDA, "Cosmetics Labeling Guide" (#2).

a site that publishes safety data on cosmetics. Here's what the site says: "Test data showed phenoxyethanol was not genotoxic nor of concern for systemic toxicity. Therefore, it was concluded to be 'safe as a cosmetic ingredient in the present practices of use and concentration,' generally < 1%."*

Now that we know phenoxyethanol is safe and used in concentrations of less than 1%, we also know that everything below it will also be less than 1%. It's possible that one or two ingredients above it might also be about 1%. I underlined *phenoxyethanol* in both lists, so you can spot it as about the 1% Line.

The amount of each ingredient is proprietary information. The items in the two columns could have some variation, or they could be the same exact same formulation made in the same vat. The consumer will never know.

What we do know is that eye cream costs a lot more than facial moisturizer, but what's the extra benefit for the extra cost? If I were in a guessing mood, I'd venture to say the benefit is less than 1%.

Eye cream is unnecessary. Use your facial moisturizer.

> *"Eye cream is unnecessary. Use your facial moisturizer."*

Serums & Essences

The term *serum* is a medical term referring to clear liquid in blood after both the cells and clotting factors are removed. Somehow, the skincare marketing world began using the word to mean something totally different. Most consumers assume the word *serum* refers to a clear water-based liquid containing skincare ingredients.

---

*   Cosmeticsinfo.org, https://cosmeticsinfo.org/ingredient/phenoxyethanol-0 (Under Safety tab)

The buzz about serums is the claim that they contain a higher concentration of certain ingredients than other facial skincare products. They may. Or they may not. Because the amount of each ingredient is not on a label, the consumer has no way of knowing the actual concentration of each ingredient. Once again, no standard definition exists for this usage of the word *serum* from the FDA, cosmetic chemists, or dermatologists.

My concern with serums is more about ingredients that they *don't* contain. Most serums do not contain ingredients that keep water from evaporating from the skin, such as petrolatum, mineral oil, or dimethicone. Without one of these types of ingredients, a product is not very effective as a moisturizer. (More on that in Chapter 8 on page 111.)

Marketing claims for serums include brightening the skin, decreasing wrinkles, and improving pigmentation. Also, serums contain ingredients with little convincing scientific evidence of their effectiveness, such as hyaluronic acid, glycolic acid, caffeine, resveratrol, peptides, and other botanicals. Without a standard definition, serums could contain anything from essential oils to green tea. All this leads to very shaky ground as to a serum's effectiveness.

This lack of scientific evidence is, surprisingly, in the manufacturers, best interest. If anyone could prove these products changed the structure or function of the skin, they would be classified as drugs. In that case, manufacturers would have to obtain FDA premarket approval at great expense. Serums are cosmetics.

FryFace Rule #3
By law, over-the-counter cosmetics, including facial moisturizers, cannot intend to change the structure or function of skin or they'd be classified as drugs.

How these products fit into a healthy skincare regimen is arbitrary. Some of them recommend application between cleansing and moisturizing. Others recommend application after moisturizing. Which one is it?

Even more confusing, the variations of serums keep growing. You can find combination serums (serum plus primer), double serums, daytime serums. and nighttime serums—taking us right back to ingredients that can tell time.

On March 16, 2020, I messaged well-respected, extremely experienced cosmetic chemist Perry Romanowski to ask, "What is the difference between a serum and an essence?"

He replied,

> Scientifically, there is no defined difference. These are marketing terms. Some serums are clear, thickened liquids. Others are emulsions in small containers. An essence can pretty much be whatever you want. Ultimately, they are all just glorified moisturizers in small containers with cosmeceutical-sounding claim ingredients.*

About ten years ago, a new skincare product arrived from Asia known as an essence. These concentrated formulas specifically target wrinkles, fine lines, and dull, uneven skin tones. This sounds like serum to me. Essence is sometimes called miracle water. The real miracle is the fact that these brilliant marketers get women to spend up to $1,500 per pound for these products.

So, what is an essence really? Depending on who you talk to—it's a serum; it's a toner; it's a moisturizer. I hear, "It's a bird; it's a plane; it's super water." And, yes, its effects are as real as

---

* Personal correspondence, used with permission.

Superman. The momentum behind all these products is not science. It's sales.

So many products, so little time, especially when standing in the aisle at the drugstore where every label says, *You're not good enough as you are.*

I have a clear solution for you:

Keep it simple. Skincare shouldn't be a full-time job or require most of your paycheck.

CHAPTER 5

Free-From Scare Tactics

Too many people have misconceptions about the FDA regulation of cosmetics in the United States. Many online and print articles base their topic matter on keyword research rather than science. They keep their analytics high by writing about issues their audience is searching for. These well-meaning writers believe they are informing the public when, in fact, they are spreading modern mythologies. Here are some myths I hear again and again.

"The FDA doesn't regulate cosmetics."

"Skincare manufacturers can do whatever they want regarding ingredients in their creams and lotions."

"Beware! Beauty products are untested and unregulated."

These statements are all false. They are false, false, and false. The US FDA regulates the cosmetics industry under the broad regulatory authority of the Federal Food, Drug, and Cosmetic Act to ensure the safety of cosmetic products. I went over this in Chapter 1 on page 13, but this topic deserves another look when we're talking about fearmongering.

The FDA does not approve cosmetics the same way they approve drugs. As a matter of fact, the FDA doesn't approve cosmetics at all. However, they do regulate them. By definition, cosmetics may claim to cleanse the body, beautify, or adorn. Cosmetics can neither intend to change the structure or function of the skin, nor can they intend to treat or prevent skin disease. Examples of cosmetics include makeup, moisturizer, perfume, and nail polish.

> *"Manufacturers have a legal responsibility to ensure their products are safe when used under customary conditions."*

Manufacturers have a legal responsibility to ensure their products are safe when used under customary conditions. They are not allowed to market adulterated or misbranded cosmetics in interstate commerce. According to the Federal Food, Drug, and Cosmetic Act, an adulterated product has one or more of the following features:

- It contains a poisonous or harmful ingredient that might harm users when the product is used as described on the product label.
- It contains a filthy, putrid, or decomposed substance.
- It is packaged, prepared, or manufactured in unsanitary conditions where it may be contaminated with microbial organisms or any substance that renders the product harmful to the consumer.
- It is packaged in a container that is composed of poisonous

or harmful substances that renders the product harmful to the user.

- It's not a hair dye but contains an unsafe color additive as determined by the FD&C Act. (Section 721(a) of the FD&C Act [21 USC. 379(a)]*

Inspectors can inspect skincare product manufacturing plants or offices without prior notice. If deemed necessary, inspections can occur on a routine basis. The FDA has the authority to:

- Restrict or ban cosmetic ingredient usage for safety reasons.
- Collect samples of cosmetic ingredients or finished products.
- Mandate warning labels on cosmetic products.
- Issue warning letters to manufacturers, packagers, or distributors.
- Seize illegal products.
- Stop unlawful activities.
- Prosecute violators of these laws.
- Collaborate with companies to implement product recalls.**

Major skincare companies know their reputation depends on safety. One incident can damage their carefully protected brand and cost them billions (with a B), so they are very careful to maintain the highest safety standards. Everyone knows this so well we take it for granted.

---

* FDA, "FDA Authority Over Cosmetics: How Cosmetics Are Not FDA-Approved, but Are FDA-Regulated."

** FDA, "Cosmetics Compliance & Enforcement."

Let's compare the safety statistics of the skincare industry with the auto industry. According to the National Safety Council, in 2017, over forty thousand people died in motor vehicle fatalities. The National Highway Traffic Safety Administration reported 1,889,000 injuries due to car accidents that same year.*

The skincare industry has approximately four hundred reported events each year.** This industry's safety record is stellar. I find it ironic that no one wants to take cars off the road, yet skincare endures a constant barrage of suspicions about safety.

> *"This industry's safety record is stellar."*

Despite this safety record, marketers often influence buying choices with free-from scare tactics, where a company implies its product is better because it does not contain certain substances.

Dose vs. Toxicity

When it comes to the safety of any substance, science refers to dose and toxicity. An adage in toxicology, the study of poisons, says the dose makes the poison. The safety of an ingredient is not related to its source, whether plant-derived or synthetic, but rather the amount of exposure or dose of the ingredient.

Water is a chemical found in nature. Water is essential for life, but drinking six liters of water in one sitting can be fatal. *Botulinum toxin* is another chemical found in nature, produced by a bacterium that grows in soil. If I inject fifty units of *botulinum toxin* type-A (commercially available as BOTOX® Cosmetic) into a woman's forehead I can paralyze the muscles,

---

* Insurance Information Institute, "Facts + Statistics: Highway safety."

** JAMA Network, "How Many Adverse Events Are Reported to FDA for Cosmetics, Personal Care?"

so she loses expression and yes, temporarily, a few wrinkles. If I inject three thousand units of the same substance, she might die from botulism.

Dose means how much of a substance the consumer comes in contact with.

Toxicity means the level at which a substance becomes damaging.

> *"Scare tactics black-list ingredients that have been proven safe when used in specified doses."*

The same is true for every chemical, whether it is a cosmetic ingredient or an approved drug. That's why cough medicine packaging and prescription bottles have recommended doses. Taken in small amounts, the substance is helpful, but an overdose has dire consequences. Scare tactics blacklist ingredients that have been proven safe when used in specified doses.

The free-from campaign is a highly effective marketing tactic. Once you become aware of it, you'll notice it everywhere. When consumers read *free-from*, they automatically assume the product is safer and better because it doesn't contain a certain ingredient. However, the ingredient may or may not be truly harmful. We're talking about marketing here, not logic or science.

One of the most popular ingredients that manufacturers target in their free-from campaigns are parabens.

Paraben-Free

To prevent contamination, all water-based moisturizers require a preservative. Without them, the vast majority of facial and body creams, lotions, and gels would become contaminated with mold, bacteria, and fungus in less than two weeks. Any water-based product will quickly become contaminated. That's a scientific fact.

Who doesn't cringe at the brown or yellow crust that accumulates on the rim of a moisturizer tube or skincare jar lid? What about the consequences of applying contaminated creams and lotions near the eyes and mouth? Preservatives are necessary to keep water-based products safe.

Parabens are a well-researched commonly used class of preservatives. They are affordable and one of the easiest ingredients to use in formulations. For consumers who love plant-derived ingredients, parabens are derived from para-hydroxybenzoic acid (PHBA), found in many fruits and vegetables like cucumbers, carrots, and blueberries.

> *"Many fruits and vegetables contain parabens."*

Of all the available preservatives, parabens have been studied the most. The Cosmetic Ingredient Review (CIR), an independent expert panel of dermatologists, toxicologists, and pharmacologists reviewed the safety of various parabens in 1984, 1986, 1995, 2009, and in 2019. They concluded that twenty different paraben ingredients are safe in cosmetics when used in approved doses.*

Keep in mind that to keep a skincare product safe, manufacturers use parabens in very tiny concentrations (less than 1%). This is true of most preservatives. One way I can get a good idea of the location of the 1% Line in an ingredient list is to simply look for a preservative.

Parabens became a media target after a poorly designed 2004 British study found parabens in breast tumor samples.** The study's author, Philippa Darbre, clarified that the study never

---

* CIR, "Amended Safety Assessment of Parabens as Used in Cosmetics."

** Darbre, "Concentrations of Parabens in Human Breast Tumours."

concluded the parabens caused the tumors. An abstract commenting on her response stated,

> ... it did not prove a direct correlation between the presence of parabens in the affected tissue and the occurrence of cancer. It also did not provide information about the possible existence of parabens in healthy tissues in the proximity of the tumor [23, 24]. Moreover, there have already been studies on the low estrogenic activity of parabens.*

Before this study was published, previous studies established that parabens can weakly mimic the natural estrogen found in the body. This, however, is also true of many foods like blueberries, carrots, flaxseed, and alfalfa sprouts.

As a result of this faulty study, advocacy groups and the media created a firestorm of fake news. Manufacturers quickly switched out their preservatives and added "Free-from Parabens" to their labels. Sales went up. In the industry this is known as consumer demand, and a new market segment was born: paraben-free skincare products.

"When you select that paraben-free product from the shelf, which preservative has replaced the parabens?"

One important question still remains. When you select a paraben-free product from the shelf, which preservative has replaced the parabens? Every water-based product must have one.

---

* Golden, "Comment on the publication by Darbre et al."

The watchdog group, Environmental Working Group (EWG) gives a Hazard Score to skincare ingredients from Best to Worst using a 10-point rating scale (with 1 being the best and 10 the worst). By their own admission, they worked with limited data when they ranked several of these preservatives.*

Here are the chemical names, followed by their Hazard Score:

- Methylparaben (a paraben), 4
- Ethylparaben (a paraben), 3
- DMDM Hydantoin, a formaldehyde-releasing preservative (not terrible, except for those with sensitive skin, eczema, or an allergy to this ingredient), 6
- Phenoxyethanol, one of the most commonly used preservatives in lieu of parabens, yet much less scrutinized than parabens, 4
- Iodopropynyl butylcarbamate, another preservative used in lieu of parabens, and much less scrutinized than parabens, 5

Many of these commonly used preservatives have worse ratings than parabens, so why don't they have free-from labels?

"Why don't other preservatives also have free-from labels?"

Are these replacements better or worse than parabens? Until someone publishes definitive studies, we cannot be sure.

If you want to go preservative-free, limit your skincare to water-free products where little, if any, preservative is necessary. That means using oil-based makeup, lotions, moisturizers, and other skincare products. However, oil-based products will also

---

* EWG, "EWG Skin Deep."

eventually become contaminated, and some have their own drawbacks. Acne-sufferers beware!

Personally, I favor parabens.

Chemical-Free

Modern mythology says that an ingredient from a plant is better, safer, and more natural. Natural and so-called chemical-free products are the fastest growing segment of the skincare industry today.

The notion of a chemical-free product is laughable because everything is made of chemicals. Glucose is the chemical name for household sugar. Sodium chloride is table salt. Acetic acid is vinegar. Dihydrogen monoxide sounds dreadful, but that's the chemical name for water.

"Everything is made of chemicals."

To debunk another common myth that if you can't pronounce the name of a chemical ingredient you shouldn't use it, try this one:

(5R)- [(1S)-1,2-Dihydroxyethyl]-3,4-dihydroxyfuran-2(5H)-one, the chemical name for ascorbic acid, or vitamin C.

Plant-based ingredients often have chemical names that are difficult to pronounce. For example, caprylic/capric triglyceride, an oil derived from coconuts, is an emollient commonly found in moisturizers. It's a skin-conditioning agent that makes the skin feel soft and smooth.

Marketing and the media have created an entire generation of chemophobes, individuals who fear chemicals. Let me reassure you, the safety standards of the skincare industry make these among the safest products you can buy. The presence of chemicals is no cause for panic.

Natural

The word *natural* on a label might imply at least some of the ingredients came from oils and extracts from herbs, plant roots, or flowers. However, plant-based ingredients have no guarantee of safety or efficacy any more than synthetic ingredients.

> *"Plant-based ingredients have no guarantee of safety or efficacy."*

Apple seeds contain amygdalin, from which the poison cyanide can be produced. Potatoes contain a deadly compound called solanine. Poison ivy is 100 percent natural, and we've all heard about Socrates who died from drinking hemlock tea, also from a plant.

Many plant-based ingredients are harmful and plenty of synthetic compounds are perfectly safe. Don't assume that because an ingredient is plant-based, it is safe. Big mistake!

Petrolatum-Free

I cringe when I see petrolatum-free on skincare product labels. Also known as petroleum jelly, petrolatum is so safe that it's used as the negative control in laboratory studies of other products. It is a scientific standard for safety.

Still, many marketing campaigns vilify petrolatum as a toxic by-product of the oil industry. United States Pharmacopeia (USP) petroleum jelly is produced in pharmaceutical-grade facilities, and that's the product you find on a retailer's shelf. Check the ingredient listing, and you'll see white petrolatum USP (100 percent).

For skeptics who believe that petroleum jelly is dangerous, please know that the FDA states that no evidence exists to support the claim that cosmetic-grade, refined petrolatum is unsafe.*

---

* Berkeley Wellness, "Is Petroleum Jelly Safe?"

This is one of the safest products on the market. (More on this in Chapter 10 on page 140.)

"Petroleum jelly is one of the safest products on the market."

If you happen to see a skincare label that says free-from petrolatum, just smile because now you have the inside story.

What You Should Avoid

Free-from campaigns use buzzwords based on market studies of words that trigger buying choices. I'd like to call your attention to some ingredients that you might want to avoid if you have certain conditions. They do not appear in any free-from campaigns, so you'll need to look at the ingredient listing.

First, check the first four to give ingredients on any bottle or jar. These few ingredients make up the bulk of the product—up to 80 or 90 percent—so look for any ingredient that might be a problem for you. For example: if you have acne watch out for isopropyl myristate, octyl stearate, or mineral oil.

Second, further down in the ingredients list, fragrance is another word to watch for. FDA regulation allows the single word *fragrance* to refer to one or more of thousands of possible ingredients, including essential oils, because labeling laws protect companies from divulging trade secrets.* Of all ingredients in skincare products, fragrance is probably Number One for causing skin reactions.**

Third, avoid products with retinoids if you suffer from sensitive skin. Retinoids can cause skin reactions in healthy skin.

---

*   FDA, "Fragrances in Cosmetics."

**   Gossens, "Contact-Allergic Reactions to Cosmetics."

They might also cause sensitivity to sunlight, making you more susceptible to sunburn. (More on this in Chapter 7 on page 95.)

The safety of each ingredient in a skincare product is certainly more important than how many ingredients are in the product. Still, with all else being equal, try to select products with fewer ingredients. Also, try to limit the number of products you use. A product with forty or fifty and sometimes up to seventy or eighty different ingredients exposes you to more risk of skin reactions, especially for someone with sensitive skin.

Check ingredients and stay with simple formulations. Remember the woman who applied an estimated 515 chemicals to her face before breakfast? Try not to be that person.

> *"Limit the number of products you use and the number of ingredients in each product."*

The only products found on skincare aisles proven to consistently improve skin health are moisturizers and sunscreen. Stick with those. Additional products such as primers, toners, astringents, facials, masks, scrubs, exfoliants, and serums are cultural pleasures. They might feel good, but little evidence shows that they are healthy for your skin. The best advice I can give you is to use fewer products.

Don't let fearmongering send you into a panic. Instead, choose a moisturizer and sunscreen that work for you and stay with them. Then, put your worries to rest. As American feminist writer Rita Mae Brown says, "Life is too short . . ."*

---

* Brown, "Life is too short to be miserable."

CHAPTER 6

Nonsense Claims

If you're not familiar with terms like *propylene glycol, triethanolamine,* or *isopropyl myristate,* you probably base your selection of skincare products on your friends' recommendations, celebrity endorsements, or merely the front label of the packaging. For most people, skincare products are a blind investment.

Skincare companies create a demand for their products with the goal of making a profit. To do this, they need to attract their ideal customer, so they engage powerful marketing departments skilled at influencing consumer buying decisions. To them, the label of a skincare product is priceless marketing real estate.

"The label of a skincare product is priceless marketing real estate."

Packaging laws ensure that skincare product labels accurately provide consumers with certain information about the product.*

---

* Federal Trade Commissions, "Fair Packaging and Labeling Act: Regulations Under Section 4 of the Fair Packaging and Labeling Act: 16 C.F.R. Part 500."

These laws state that the front panel of a package must identify the product and the amount in the dispenser, so buyers can compare prices. Labels must also show the manufacturer, distributor, and the ingredient listing. Certain ingredients require warning panels. This information is all valid and valuable.

Unfortunately, along with the useful information, some labels are also studded with senseless jargon. The objective: to convince the buyer that this product offers an immediate solution for some skincare challenge. That challenge might be real, or it might be completely made up.

For example, the word *rejuvenate* often appears on skincare labels. The implied message to the consumer: everyone should renew his or her skin. However, no over-the-counter moisturizer makes the skin new again. The skin does that all on its own every twenty-eight days. Once a month the outer layer of skin completely refreshes itself.

In previous chapters, I covered many examples of marketing lingo similar to this example. To prompt a buying decision, product labels use words with high emotional impact and little meaning, such as:

- Terms that feed off of our fears about getting older, such as *anti-aging*, even though science has yet to find a single ingredient that can reverse the aging process.
- In 2017, *Allure* magazine decided to stop using the term *anti-aging*: "With that in mind, and starting with this issue, we are making a resolution to stop using the term 'anti-aging.' Whether we know it or not, we're subtly reinforcing the message that aging is a condition we need to battle—think anti-anxiety meds, antivirus software, or antifungal spray."*

---

* Lee, *"Allure* Magazine Will No Longer Use the Term "Anti-Aging."

- Terms that contribute to the unfortunate cultural belief that youth is equal to beauty, such as *age-defying*.
- Phrases used out of context to stretch the limits of reality by describing something that doesn't even apply to the skin such as polishing, detoxifying, or nourishing. Good words when used properly, they make absolutely no sense when pertaining to skin.
- Terminology that seems to add legitimacy to the product but has little or no true value, like *dermatologist tested*.

Marketing buzzwords on skincare product labels are ingenious, convincing, and very creative. They are psychologically designed to sway the consumer's choice about whether to buy the product or not.

Legally, the manufacturer must be in compliance with labeling laws, properly identify the contents of the package, and use wording consumers can understand. Beyond that, when it comes to the verbiage on cosmetic labels, anything else is game. The possibilities for nonsense claims are endless. Here are a few of them:

Stem Cells

One of the trendiest buzzwords found on skincare product labels today is stem cells. Cosmetic products that are sitting on drugstore shelves do not contain living stem cells. I can say this with complete confidence because stem cells cannot survive in skincare emulsions. They require an environment that is pH-balanced at a certain temperature. Retail cosmetic lotions, creams, serums, or gels do not provide these conditions. Aside from that, moisturizers contain preservatives, which kill all living organisms, including stem cells.

> *"Moisturizers contain preservatives which kill all living organisms, including stem cells."*

Most plant and animal cells have a given purpose. For example, plants have leaf cells and root cells while animals have nerve cells and muscle cells. Stem cells can come from either plants or animals. They are unique because they don't have one specific purpose. These cells are highly adaptable and can either divide to become more stem cells, or they can develop a purpose, such as becoming a leaf cell and dividing to create more leaf cells.

Ingredient manufacturers use plant stem cells by genetically programming them to produce plant-based compounds. For example, arbutin is a compound successfully produced from the bearberry plant using stem cell technology. In the laboratory, arbutin has been shown to slow pigment formation, and therefore, is commonly added to cosmetics marketed as dark-spot removers.*

The true benefit of stem cell technology does not come from adding stem cells to skincare products as an ingredient. The true benefit comes from stem-cell factories that produce high quality, plant-based ingredients in controlled concentrations.

Plant extracts produced from stem cells in sterile conditions have no risk of contamination from organisms or pesticide exposure. In the laboratory, they don't have to deal with variations of soil conditions and environmental factors from weather and changing seasons. Major challenges when using plant-based materials include controlling purity and concentration. When produced from stem cells, however, the result is a cleaner, more consistent ingredient, and most importantly, a more standardized final product.

Unfortunately, producing plant extracts via stem cells is an expensive proposition. The process has potential, but thus far the research doesn't verify the effectiveness of these extracts or the safety of these techniques for public use.

---

* Trehan, "Plant stem cells in cosmetics: current trends and future directions."

Stem cells are not the new Fountain of Youth. Don't believe the buzz.

Hypoallergenic

When a cosmetics label contains the term *hypoallergenic*, the manufacturer wants you to believe that their product is less likely to cause an allergic reaction than non-hypoallergenic products. Without comparison testing with published results, the term hypoallergenic has very little meaning and, therefore, little value.

No single test can guarantee a consumer will be safe from an allergic reaction after using any particular product. No federal guidelines exist for this kind of testing. In fact, the term hypoallergenic has no government-required testing protocol. The manufacturer might have tested the product on a small number of subjects, but they might have done no testing at all.

Major internationally and nationally recognized brands do some sort of product testing as part of their safety analysis, and some testing is better than none at all. That's one reason I recommend you purchase products from the larger reputable manufacturers. It's possible that they tested their wares on thirty subjects or, if the budget allows, maybe one hundred subjects. However, you and I have no way to be sure of the level of testing done on any particular product.

Ironically, products labeled hypoallergenic often contain at least one ingredient, usually a preservative, known to cause skin reactions, especially for people with sensitive skin. The FDA does not require manufacturers of skincare products to submit substantiation of their hypoallergenic claims before going to market. Therefore, the term has very little meaning.

> *"Products labeled hypoallergenic often contain at least one ingredient known to cause skin reactions."*

Despite the lack of evidence, hypoallergenic is an extremely effective marketing term, frequently found on the front label of skincare products. When using a new product, I recommend you first test it on your forearm or behind your ear before using it on large areas of the skin. However, even pre-testing is no absolute guarantee that a skin reaction won't occur when you use the product regularly.

Non-Comedogenic

The term *non-comedogenic* on the label implies that the product was specifically formulated, so it won't cause blocked pores, also called comedones, such as blackheads or whiteheads. This term is most appealing to individuals with oily or acne-prone skin who are concerned that the product might cause a breakout. The FDA does not define the term, nor does it declare which ingredients to exclude from a product to qualify as non-comedogenic.

Truth is, no federal standard, guideline, or testing protocol guarantees that the user will have a clear complexion after using a product. No independent organization can affirm whether or not a product is non-comedogenic.

> *"No independent organization can affirm whether or not a product is non-comedogenic."*

During product development, many reputable companies test to see whether a formulation will trigger breakouts, but again, they are not required to. The law requires that they make sure their products are safe when used in a customary manner and when used according to the directions on the label.

Skin is highly individual. What might cause a breakout in one person might not affect another at all. Standardizing any particular ingredient as non-comedogenic is a challenge.

Does the term non-comedogenic have any value? Although this term has no regulatory standards, many reputable manufacturers design their formulations with acne-prone individuals in mind, as well as those who have excessively oily skin. These individuals might find the term helpful when selecting products, but it's not an absolute guarantee of clear skin. Non-comedogenic is yet another unverifiable marketing term found on skincare product labels.

Dermatologist Tested

One of my favorite nonsense claims found on skincare product labels is *dermatologist tested*. These words imply that at least one dermatologist tested the product. This dermatologist might have applied the product to some part of a body—perhaps his or her own—for a period of time, or maybe just once. We don't know if the dermatologist has a financial interest in the product, or if the tester is an individual or a group of dermatologists. Who knows if the product was actually tested at all?

No federal guideline or standard definition exists for this meaningless buzzword.

Once again, I recommend that you purchase skincare products from major manufacturers. My reasons include: (1) Larger companies have the resources to test and produce safe, consistent products; (2) they have long-standing reputations at stake, a powerful motivator to keep their customers safe; and (3) many of them are members of the Personal Care Products Council (PCPC), a leading national trade organization committed to producing quality products.

Nourishing

Sometimes I think the people who think up these skincare ads chose to go into creative fields because they didn't do well in biology. These ads seem to confuse body parts and their functions on a regular basis.

For example, advertisements often imply that your skin needs to breathe. Actually, your lungs do that. Skin does not take in oxygen or give off carbon dioxide. Others describe how a certain product detoxes the skin, but the liver, kidneys, and gastrointestinal tract have that function covered. Exactly which toxins do these marketing experts believe skin excretes? I can't name one.

Jargon such as *nourishing* encourages consumers to believe that they need to feed the skin, and their product will provide food. This is medical nonsense. When applied on the surface of the skin, skincare products come in contact with the outer fifteen to twenty layers of nonliving cells. Nourishing dead tissue is medically impossible. In lower skin layers that are living, skin receives nourishment from its blood supply.

"Nourishing dead tissue is medically impossible."

Healthy skin parallels a healthy body. Nourished skin is the result of a nutritious diet rich in fruits, vegetables, lean protein, and healthy carbs, as well as adequate sleep and exercise. Science also demonstrates that skin health improves when we avoid stressors like smoking and ultraviolet light. None of these healthy behaviors involve rubbing on a nourishing cream, lotion, or gel.

The word *nourish* is very creative, yet senseless, marketing-speak.

Firming

Have you ever gone up to a friend and said, "Wow, your skin looks so firm"?

What does firm skin look like? And how do you measure firm skin? Is a machine or device available to measure skin firmness?

If your skin isn't firm, I assume that means it's wrinkled or sagging. Does the marketing lingo on that firming cream imply that this skincare product can eliminate wrinkles or lift sagging skin? As a cosmetic, the product cannot intend to change your skin, or it would be classified as a drug and require FDA approval. I can only assume that the word *firm* in firming cream implies hydration, which means plumping up with water. Basically, firming creams are simply moisturizers.

> *"Firming creams are simply moisturizers."*

Either way, don't waste your money on a firming cream. This term is meaningless slanguage.

Polishing

The list of things we must do to have the healthiest skin seems to keep growing. Clean it. Scrub it. Hydrate it. Exfoliate it. Tone it. Firm it. Unclog it. Rest it. Stimulate it. Detox it. And, now this, polish it. I laughed hysterically when I saw a TV commercial advertising skin polish. Like a car, make it shine.

But wait. We don't want it to shine. Isn't that why we supposedly need a toner?

What next? Maybe ads that promote adding a wax or a veneer to the skin? Never mind, that won't work because the skin won't be able to breathe.

Maybe I should take a breath because I'm getting carried away.

These crazy ideas don't stop. Could it be, just maybe, your skin is perfect the way it is? Is it conceivable that your skin is functioning just the way it should and has absolutely no need for this new skin polish? Polishing skin belongs at the top of the list of marketing foolishness.

*"Polishing skin belongs at the top of the list
of marketing foolishness."*

The nonsense claims go on and on. They vigorously fuel my passion to speak the truth and empower women with solid, verifiable information. The most common marketing terminology on facial skincare products today involves aging. Age-related marketing is so abundant, so demeaning, and so ageist that I devoted the entire next chapter to this topic.

CHAPTER 7

Anti-Aging
Fairy Tales

Today, the quest for youth is an epidemic. Medical researchers continue to advance our understanding of how our bodies change as we mature, yet science has not found a single ingredient or product that halts or reverses aging. Still, skincare aisles overflow with "anti-aging" creams and lotions.

My first question is always: Why do you want to defy your age? If you've had the good fortune to live long enough to celebrate many milestones and experience the joys of seeing new generations among your family and friends, consider yourself fortunate. A long life is a tremendous blessing of priceless value.

Going back to the science, the majority of "anti-aging" cosmetic creams have formulations similar to facial moisturizers with marketing tool ingredients added. These ingredients have one main purpose: to satisfy the age-reversing claims on the product label.

> *"Marketing tool ingredients have one main purpose: to satisfy the age-reversing claims on the product label."*

Green tea extract is a good example. Manufacturers add green tea extract to a product to back up their claim that the product has "anti-aging" properties. First of all, no science shows that green tea extract rolls back the clock on skin aging. Second, if the extract is intended to reverse aging, the product must be classified as a drug. Otherwise, its presence on the cosmetic skincare aisle is illegal. The same is true for resveratrol, vitamin C, vitamin E, hyaluronic acid, and on and on.

The FDA does not approve individual cosmetic products. Cosmetics like anti-aging creams are luxury items designed to make the user feel good, despite the fact that they cannot intend to have a lasting impact on the skin. Cosmetic skincare companies take poetic license and use an array of clever formulating tactics to declare certain ingredients as anti-aging. They may add a negligible amount of one or more of these marketing tool ingredients to a moisturizer, paste the word *anti-aging* on the label, and charge a higher price point. All in an attempt to increase sales, the true measure of a product's success.

That's why I call these ingredients marketing tools. In my opinion, manufacturers add them simply to validate the marketing. Regardless of what they might claim, the fact remains that science has yet to find a single ingredient or product that can halt or reverse aging.

We see facial creams marketed for mature skin simply to target an older consumer base, the same way baby moisturizers target the baby market. The contents of these bottles or jars might very well come from the same vat.

What could possibly validate a claim that a facial cream is for mature skin?

- At what age does skin become mature? Fifty, sixty, seventy years? Some people would say thirty-five. Who makes that judgment?
- How does a mature-skin formulation perform differently than a regular formulation?
- Do ingredients really perform differently on a twenty-year-old face than they do on a seventy-year-old face?

Healthy skin does not have a time signature. A quality moisturizer is effective whether the consumer is seventeen or seventy-seven. Ingredients don't tell time, and they don't recognize age.

"Healthy skin does not have a time signature."

Here are some types of ingredients frequently used to validate anti-aging marketing claims.

Antioxidants

The Free Radical Theory of Aging is one of many aging theories. While not popular with most reputable evolutionary biologists,* this theory does get a lot of attention in the cosmetic industry. Why? It provides a list of ingredients, namely antioxidants, to boost sales. And sell they do, to the tune of a $4-billion-per-year antioxidant market in the US alone.**

---

* American Federation of Aging Research, "Theories of Aging."

** Prasad, "Global Antioxidants Market."

The skincare industry is obsessed with antioxidants. If you listen to the ads and reviews, antioxidants are a modern miracle. They protect the skin and prevent skin cancer. They make you look younger. They seem to do everything. Although no definitive science proves antioxidants reverse the aging process, marketing experts constantly refer to antioxidants as the good guys.

> *"No definitive science proves that antioxidants reverse the aging process."*

Most consumers aren't even sure what antioxidants are. When I ask people for a definition, they usually say, "They're found in blueberries."

I like to explain antioxidants with a simple comparison. Everyone knows flammable items are substances that can catch fire, such as paper, wood, gasoline, hand sanitizer, and rubbing alcohol. Flammables have one thing in common: they can burn.

Antioxidants are a group of compounds that share one simple property: they can neutralize oxidants, also known as free radicals. Vitamin C, resveratrol, coenzyme Q, niacinamide, green tea extract, and vitamin E are all examples of antioxidants that can be taken by mouth. The skincare industry mixes these substances into creams and lotions.

Our bodies need antioxidants because they prevent damage to cells. Yet, how many do we need? What kinds do we need? Does applying antioxidants to the skin have any real benefit?

Just as the word *flammable* describes a wide variety of items, the broad term *antioxidants* also includes a wide variety of substances that perform various functions. When building a home, a builder needs all kinds of tools: hammers, saws, power drills, screwdrivers, and more. Showing up at the job site with a toolbox filled with hammers isn't going to help much. Similarly, applying one type of antioxidant to the skin isn't necessarily beneficial either.

> *"Applying one type of antioxidant to the skin isn't necessarily beneficial."*

If antioxidants are the good guys, then oxidants must be the bad guys, right? Oxidants or free radicals are unstable oxygen molecules that cause cell death. They increase with sunlight, tobacco usage, and alcohol consumption. Fact is, oxidants are a by-product of breathing. We all make them. They are an unavoidable part of life.

Are free radicals really the bad guys? I don't think so. They increase with exercise. The medical community promotes exercise as a beneficial and integral part of a healthy lifestyle. Substantial scientific evidence backs this up.

Oxidants are a double-edged sword. Science shows free radicals to be necessary for wound healing.* The immune system needs free radicals to defend our bodies from illness and infection. The same free radicals that destroy healthy cells also destroy unhealthy cells to help us heal, overcome infections, and fight cancer.

> *"Free radicals speed healing, overcome infections, and fight cancer."*

While antioxidants have their benefits, plenty of evidence confirms too many can be harmful.** The human body is in a

---

* Xu, "C. elegans epidermal wounding induces a mitochondrial ROS burst that promotes wound repair."

** National Cancer Institute, "Alpha-Tocopherol, Beta-Carotene Cancer Prevention (ATBC) Study."

battle of good versus evil every second of every minute of every day. We constantly maintain a delicate balance of antioxidants and free radicals, including in our skin. In other words, we need both.

Drugstore shelves are full of "anti-aging" creams that tell a tantalizing fairy tale about restoring more youthful skin with antioxidants. It's brilliant marketing. It works. However, science does not prove that antioxidants reverse the aging process.

Antioxidants are unstable. They quickly become deactivated in the presence of light and oxygen. This explains why many skincare products formulated with antioxidants come in opaque bottles and metal tubes. Keeping them active in formulated creams or lotions is a challenge. If they survive the formulation process, viable antioxidants quickly lose their effectiveness once applied to the skin where they are exposed to light and oxygen.

> *"Keeping antioxidants active in formulated creams or lotions is a challenge."*

Certain antioxidants have a minimal sun-protection effect on nonliving cells on the skin's surface.* However, the top layer isn't where skin wrinkling or the predominance of aging occurs. Antioxidants cannot penetrate deeply enough at a high enough concentration to impact wrinkles.

In order to do so, enough antioxidant would have to penetrate through fifteen to twenty layers of nonliving cells, down through an additional fifty to sixty layers of living epidermal cells, through a basement membrane, and further into the second

---

* Al-Niaimi, "Topical Vitamin C and the Skin: Mechanisms of Action and Clinical Applications."

layer of skin to reach the structural proteins that keep the skin looking supple and youthful.

To put it simply, antioxidants constantly decay in formulations. Even if they did survive, they can't adequately penetrate the skin anyway.

"Antioxidants can't adequately penetrate the skin."

Over-the-counter antioxidant-containing anti-aging, anti-wrinkle, age-defying creams have one main benefit: they increase water content of the skin. That's what well-formulated moisturizers do—without antioxidants, without marketing hype, or silly anti-aging fairy tales.

Increasing the water content of skin temporarily improves the appearance of fine lines. As for actual wrinkle improvement, not so much. Moisturizers, even well-formulated ones, cannot remove wrinkles from your face.

Retinoids

I'm often asked about anti-wrinkle products that contain retinoids, a class of vitamin A compounds that are also antioxidants. Many dermatologists and other skincare experts consider retinoids the gold standard anti-wrinkle superstar ingredients. I disagree.

Based on my thirty years of experience, I tell my patients to weigh the benefits of a product against the disadvantages before they buy. What are the side effects, the limitations, and the cost? I call this the benefit-risk ratio. When the benefit is great and the risk is low, the product is a good choice.

"When the benefit is great and the risk is low,
the product is a good choice."

This concept applies to many life choices. For example, we all know the benefits of driving a car. We gain independence, flexibility of time, the ability to travel further distances compared to walking or biking and, for many, a relaxing activity. Driving also introduces the risk of getting into a car accident, although seatbelts and safe speeds minimize that risk. When the benefit is high and the risk is low, we choose to drive.

In the event of bad weather, the risk becomes greater. We might choose to stay at home until the sun comes out and the risk is lower. Most of us make these choices with little conscious thought.

Back to the retinoids, the benefit-risk ratio of using topical retinoids is low with little benefit and significant risk. When you factor in the high cost, retinoids do not seem to be a good choice.

Let's consider tretinoin, a retinoid that requires a prescription. Let me clarify that in this writing I am referring to retinoid therapy used for anti-aging treatment only. Topical creams, ointments, and gels containing tretinoin are also approved by the FDA to treat acne, a true medical condition. The benefits and risks to be considered when selecting medication to treat a potentially scarring inflammation are very different from those of a cosmetic concern.

The products I refer to here are tretinoin products approved for mitigation or lessening of fine facial wrinkles. Meaning, it is approved as an adjuvant therapy, a complementary ingredient, for users who follow a comprehensive sun protection program and avoid direct sunlight exposure. In other words, this product helps reduce fine lines for people who also avoid the sun, cover up with hats and clothing, and apply lots of sunscreen while outdoors.

Laboratory science shows that retinoids like tretinoin have a positive effect on gene arrangement and collagen production.

However, these studies show few cosmetic benefits with statistically significant clinical results to back them up.

Renova® is an FDA-approved tretinoin cream for fine wrinkles. The package insert for Renova® clearly states: "RENOVA® (tretinoin cream) 0.02% DOES NOT ELIMINATE WRINKLES, REPAIR SUN-DAMAGED SKIN, REVERSE PHOTOAGING, or RESTORE MORE YOUTHFUL or YOUNGER SKIN."*

The insert contains clinical data from five clinical trials. Only twenty-eight of 279 participants, or 10 percent of those who applied tretinoin and sunscreen had moderate improvement in fine wrinkles. Of the remaining 251 participants, 212 showed mild or minimal improvement, no change, or even a worsening of the skin. All of these participants had lighter skin. In a similar study of darker-skinned individuals, participants fared worse than those who only used sun protection.

Another prescription retinoid, AVAGE® Cream, contains tazarotene which is also approved by the FDA with similar indications as tretinoin as described above. The AVAGE® prescription package insert reads,

Limitations of Use:

- Does not eliminate or prevent wrinkles or restore more youthful skin.
- Does not repair sun damaged skin or reverse photoaging.
- Safety and effectiveness for the prevention or treatment of actinic keratoses, skin neoplasms, or lentigo maligna have not been established.**

---

*   FDA, "RENOVA (TRETINOIN CREAM 0.02%)."

**   FDA, "Avage and Tazorac Labeling."

Again, only a small percentage of users saw moderate improvement.

Keep in mind, these studies involved prescription-strength retinoids which are magnitudes stronger than retinoids found in over-the-counter products.

I have prescribed topical retinoids to hundreds, maybe thousands, of patients who requested this popular therapy with the hopes of minimizing their facial wrinkles, despite knowing that moderate improvement is seen in only 10 percent of users based on my experience and clinical studies. Eighty to ninety percent of them experienced initial flaking, burning, or irritation. For some, these uncomfortable side effects lessened over time, but far too many continued to have side effects despite applying moisturizers several times a day. I was among those who had persistent irritation and redness for as long as I used the product.

About 90 percent of my patients who attempted anti-wrinkle retinoid therapy experienced little benefit and after many months discontinued therapy. Retinoids have a high potential for side effects, need consistent and diligent sun avoidance, and cost up to $500 per tube. In my opinion, prescription retinoids have a low benefit-risk ratio.

Over-the-counter cosmetic retinoids, like retinol, are exponentially less effective than their prescription counterparts. While side effects are more moderate, some people still experience irritation and burning, especially those with eczema and sensitive skin.

All retinoid creams may increase sensitivity to sunlight and increase the chance of sunburn. Users must avoid direct sun exposure and wear protective clothing, hats, and liberal amounts of sunscreen. All this for meager, if any, results. Based on thirty years of dermatology practice, the scientific literature, and my personal experience with both prescription and over-the-counter vitamin A compounds, retinoids have a low benefit-risk ratio and are not a good choice for reducing wrinkles.

> *"The low benefit-risk ratio makes retinoids a poor buying choice."*

Since clinical evidence shows little proof that topical retinoids are effective anti-wrinkle creams, I suggest using a well-formulated moisturizer if your skin is dry and apply sunscreen daily. (More on the full benefits of sunscreen in Chapter 9 on page 115.)

Hyaluronic Acid

Hyaluronic acid is another common ingredient in "anti-aging" skincare products. I love this ingredient, but not for the reason you might think.

Over-the-counter anti-wrinkle products decrease the appearance of fine lines by increasing water content in the skin. Imagine a wrinkled raisin. Pump water into it, and *voilà*, you have a grape! Well, sort of. The surface becomes a bit smoother, at least temporarily. Does this description fulfill the meaning of *anti-wrinkle*? Does the raisin look exactly like a fresh grape? Not so much.

> *"Hyaluronic acid is a very effective ingredient in moisturizers."*

Hyaluronic acid is a major component of the body's connective tissue, bones, cartilage, tendons, and ligaments. Almost half of the body's hyaluronic acid is found in the skin.

When not bound to other molecules, hyaluronic acid binds to large amounts of water, many times its weight. Hyaluronic acid is a very effective ingredient in moisturizers because it attracts water to the skin's surface. Combined with a protective ingredient such as dimethicone or petrolatum to prevent water from evaporating into the environment, hyaluronic acid is a key ingredient in some of the most effective topical moisturizers.

However, the hyaluronic acid molecule is massive. Trying to push it down into the skin where wrinkles form is like trying to drive a tractor trailer through the door of a coffee shop. I recently saw a marketing campaign promoting low molecular weight hyaluronic acid that supposedly penetrates the skin, but neither science nor clinical evidence consistently proves this claim. Any claims that topical hyaluronic acid can penetrate the skin deeply enough to reverse signs of aging is pure marketing hype.

> *"Claims that topical hyaluronic acid can penetrate the skin deeply enough to reverse signs of aging is pure marketing hype."*

Besides, if this ingredient or any other actually changes the skin, it must be classified as . . . you know this . . . a drug!

The term *anti-aging* is the most brilliant marketing slogan, *ever*! It consumes us. However, the more we try, the more we fail.

> *"The term anti-aging is the most brilliant marketing slogan, ever!"*

We buy and keep on buying. When a $50-per-ounce product doesn't work, we buy an $80 product. We follow trends and read the latest product reviews. When we pay $150 per ounce, we are spending $2,400 per pound, and some will keep going, spending up to $8,000 per pound—all too often with unfulfilled expectations. To put these costs into perspective, you can purchase grass-fed local filet mignon for $40 per pound.

Can you think of any perishable item that you would even consider spending $8,000 per pound on? Let alone, on a product that fails to show results over and over again? And one that, by law, cannot intend to change the actual structure of the skin? This defies sensible thinking, and yet I see it happening far too often.

We fight. We fight crepiness, sagging, thinning, and darkening. We fight free radicals. Most of all, we fight wrinkles.

We stretch the limits of logic. We go after ingredients *du jour* such as bee venom, snail slime, or nightingale poop. We try serums with an enchanting tea extract or peptide. We smear on black charcoal creams and facial foams with placenta from Australia. All of this effort and expense with little or no evidence to show that they really work.

We continue to fight the wrinkle. We change our behavior. Some say sleeping on your back prevents wrinkles—as if anyone has control once they've fallen sound asleep. Most people rotate fifteen to fifty times an hour in deep sleep. Of course, you could always tie yourself down.

We buy fad products. Silk pillowcases are said to prevent facial wrinkles by helping skin retain moisture and minimize chemical exposure, though from what chemicals I do not know.

We tape our foreheads before bed to prevent frown lines and do facial exercises to prevent sagging. I cannot find a single legitimate study to back up the benefits of these routines. Don't expect healthier skin from using them.

My conclusion: Like unicorns, mermaids, and tooth fairies, anti-wrinkle creams and other anti-aging products are fairy tales. We love to believe in them, but little science proves that any of them are real.

CHAPTER 8

What Moisturizers Really Do

Facial creams, night creams, eye creams, body lotions, firming and "anti-aging" creams, age-defying potions, many OTC creams marketed to improve eczema, psoriasis, or diabetic skin, products to smooth cracks on fingertips and heels, lip balms, and products to improve dry skin—all have one thing in common: All are moisturizers. Some are more effective than others.

Well-controlled studies on moisturizer ingredients are few and far between. Labels list ingredients with long chemical names. Fear-based statements in the media, "new discoveries" that have no basis in science, the exaggerated drive for all-natural products and flashy celebrity endorsements—all create a lot of noise. I understand why consumers stay confused and overwhelmed.

People have preferences about whether they like their moisturizer thick or thin, clear or opaque, scented or unscented, and they often have a preferred type of dispenser. An often-overlooked factor in a buying decision is whether the moisturizer actually supports healthy skin. Unless you have some education about skincare, you might assume all do. However, that's not the case. Even if a cream or lotion makes your skin look smoother and feel softer, only testing determines whether a product supports healthy skin by increasing its water content.

> *"Only testing determines whether a product supports healthy skin by increasing its water content."*

Medical literature is full of studies that show the benefits of increasing water content of skin and improving the skin's water barrier function.

Dermatologists agree that effective moisturizers:

- Maintain healthy skin.
- Relieve dryness.
- Improve many skin conditions, such as eczema and atopic dermatitis.
- Diminish the discomforts of the skin's feeling tight, itching, stinging, and pain.
- Enhance skin appearance.
- Improve self-esteem.

While most dermatologists have a basic knowledge of a handful of common ingredients, many don't fully understand how moisturizers are formulated or how they come to market.

This information is not a major part of the dermatology residency curriculum.

The Word *Moisturizer* Is a Misnomer

The word *moisturizer* has no standardized definition—not among dermatologists nor within the skincare industry. In fact, moisturizer is a marketing term without any medical or scientific origin. It falls into the same category as Chinese Checkers—which aren't a form of checkers, nor are they from China—and jellyfish that aren't really fish. Neither are starfish, for that matter.

> *"The word moisturizer is a marketing term."*

Moisturizer is actually a misnomer because it leads people to assume that moisturizers add water to the skin. They don't. The skin does that all on its own by pulling water from within the body. An effective moisturizer supports the skin barrier and slows down water loss from the top-most layer of the skin. This allows the skin to hydrate itself from within and repair the natural moisture barrier.

The skin absorbs little water from outside, and that's a good thing. Otherwise, we'd swell up like a sponge whenever we take a shower or dip into the pool. Although imperfect, skin is a brilliant series of layered cells with each cell wrapped in water-resistant fat. It makes us virtually waterproof by preventing water from both entering and leaving the body.

> *"An effective moisturizer supports the skin barrier by slowing down water loss from the skin."*

By decreasing the amount of water loss, not only does the skin look and feel softer, but it can also do a better job protecting us from bacteria, parasites, fungus, viruses, heat, and ultraviolet rays from the sun. Conditions like atopic dermatitis, seborrheic dermatitis, psoriasis, and acne all improve when skin is well hydrated.*

The Basic Recipe

Whether they are facial lotions, body lotions, eye creams, foot creams, hand creams, night creams, or "anti-aging" lotions—the majority of moisturizers have the same fundamental recipe.

> *"The majority of moisturizers have the same fundamental recipe."*

When I speak on this topic, I use the analogy of a basic yellow cake recipe that calls for flour, sugar, baking powder, eggs, butter, milk, salt, and vanilla. Each of these ingredients serves a specific function.

- Flour: The foundational structure for the cake comes from flour. I use white flour, but almond flour or whole wheat would also work.
- Sugar: I prefer granulated sugar as the sweetener, but I could use a sugar substitute or brown sugar.
- Baking powder: The rising ingredient in my recipe is baking powder, but baking soda and yeast also cause rising.
- Eggs: Eggs hold the cake together and so do soaked chia seeds.
- Butter: Fat provides a smooth texture and moisture to

---

* Purnamawati, "The Role of Moisturizers in Addressing Various Kinds of Dermatitis: A Review," 75-87.

the cake. I prefer real butter but some use shortening, oil, or margarine.

- Milk: The liquid could be 2% milk, evaporated milk, or water to transform the dry ingredients into a batter.
- Salt: As an accent flavoring, pink Himalayan salt, sea salt, or the white stuff in the round blue box would all work.
- Vanilla: The flavoring could also be cocoa or rum flavoring. Orange juice could serve as both moisture and flavoring.
- Added features: Extra fixings such as bananas, chocolate chips, or nuts would make the cake unique. If I were selling my cakes, I'd call these additional items marketing ingredients.

Whatever your choices, the basic yellow cake recipe (the formulation) stays the same. This concept holds true for formulated moisturizers. The overwhelming majority of over-the-counter moisturizers are water based and have a comparable recipe:

- Water: Liquid where all the other ingredients are dissolved.
- Occlusives: Create a film barrier to keep water from evaporating.
- Humectants: Draw water up to the skin's surface.
- Emollients: Make the skin feel soft.
- Emulsifiers: Keep ingredients from separating.
- Thickeners: Give the product consistency.
- Preservatives: Prevent bacterial and fungal overgrowth.
- Fragrances: Make it smell good.

Here's what each of these ingredient types contributes to the moisturizer.

Water

The majority of moisturizing lotions and creams contain 60 to 80 percent water, the solvent in which all the other ingredients are blended. Since water has the highest percentage in the formulation, it's often the first item on the ingredient list.

> *"The majority of moisturizing lotions and creams contain 60 to 80 percent water."*

Occlusives

By creating a barrier on the skin's surface, occlusives prevent water from evaporating. The most common occlusive in skincare products today is petrolatum. It is often high up on the ingredient list.

I might consider petrolatum the perfect occlusive if it weren't so greasy. Although not as effective as petrolatum, many other waxy and fatty substances that aren't as greasy prevent water evaporation in moisturizer formulations, including cetyl alcohol (from palm oil or coconut oil), lanolin (from sheep's wool) or mineral oil. These are all oil-based substances.

Oil-free moisturizers often use a synthetic silicone occlusive like dimethicone to minimize the greasy feel. Silicones do not prevent water evaporation as effectively as petroleum jelly. People with oily skin who don't need as much water-barrier support do well with oil-free products. Reputable manufacturers often combine various occlusives to create a moisture barrier that is both effective and pleasant to the consumer.

Humectants

Humectants are water magnets. They draw water from the deeper layers of skin to the surface and also pull water from the air on very humid days. Commonly used humectants in over-the-counter skincare products include glycerin, sorbitol, propylene glycol, and hyaluronic acid.

Applying humectants alone, especially on damaged skin, can increase water loss and result in drier skin. The most effective moisturizers contain both occlusives and humectants. Humectants draw water to the skin's surface, and occlusives keep the water from evaporating.

Emollients

Emollients are smoothing ingredients that fill in between dry skin flakes and scales. They make your skin feel soft. Some commonly used emollients are mineral oil, shea butter, dimethicone (yes, the same ingredient that also serves as an occlusive), and plant oils such as coconut oil.

Emulsifiers

Any moisturizer that contains both water and oil components needs an ingredient to keep them from separating. Emulsifiers do just that. Without emulsifiers, the oils create a layer on the top of the bottle or jar, and the water-soluble ingredients stay in a layer below, much like oil and vinegar dressing. Laureth-4 and polysorbates are common emulsifiers.

Thickeners

Few consumers want a moisturizer that splashes onto their hands like water. Thickeners provide a consistency most people like and help keep the product where they need it. Thickeners also help the product remain stable. Frequently used thickeners include carbomer and cetyl alcohol.

Preservatives

No one is happy to find green mold or black bacteria in their jar of face cream. Without preservatives, bacterial and fungal overgrowth occurs in every water-based product within two weeks. I mentioned preservatives before in our discussion about parabens on page 71. Other examples of commonly used preservatives are phenoxyethanol and DMDM hydantoin.

Fragrances

Smell is the most distinguishing characteristic of any skincare product and also the most important to consumers. I often see women on skincare aisles flipping open product caps and raising the tube to their noses in an attempt to smell the moisturizer before they buy it. As a result, manufacturers conduct detailed marketing studies to see which fragrance combinations are most attractive to customers. Their signature smells become an integral part of the company's trademarked branding.

> *"Fragrance is a blanket term that can refer to one or a combination of ingredients without revealing what they are."*

In the ingredients listing, fragrances might be listed as fragrance, flavor, parfum, or by listing the name of one or more essential oil. By law, the word fragrance in an ingredient listing is a blanket term that can refer to one or a combination of ingredients without revealing what they are. The FDA considers fragrance mixtures to be proprietary trade secrets.

Although scent has the biggest impact on sales, fragrances are the most common causes of allergic skin reactions. I recommend individuals with sensitive skin or allergic tendencies to select products labeled fragrance-free. Doing so helps minimize the chances of a skin reaction. However, even with fragrance-free on the label, fragrances might still be present in the product because some are used for purposes other than smell. For example, essential oils create a pleasant smell but are also emollients.

Benzyl alcohol is a fragrance, but sometimes it might take the role of a preservative in a formulation.

> *"Even with fragrance-free on the label,*
> *fragrances might still be present in the product*
> *because some are used for purposes other than smell."*

Unscented products might add masking fragrances to block unpleasant odors caused by other ingredients. If you see *unscented* on a label, it means the product has no smell. It does not mean the absence of fragrances.

Sometimes manufacturers add certain fragrances because consumers believe products with certain scents are more effective. For example, some people think a shampoo with menthol is better to relieve itchy symptoms—even though this is not necessarily so.

Manufacturers consider many factors when they choose ingredients to put into their formulations. Is the product a liquid, cream, or gel? Clear or opaque? Can one ingredient fulfill more than one role? For example, dimethicone and cetyl alcohol are both occlusives and emollients. Some preservatives have a pleasant fragrance, so they can serve two roles. Hundreds of ingredients create millions of possible combinations.

The ingredients a manufacturer chooses make all the difference in the effectiveness of their product. Reputable manufacturers have the advantage of research and development departments filled with teams of cosmetic chemists well versed in what each ingredient does. Consumers do not have that information, so they often misunderstand the purpose and characteristics of some ingredients.

Misunderstood Ingredients

A great example of a misunderstood ingredient in skincare products is alcohol. Many consumers incorrectly believe that all alcohols dry and irritate the skin. Alcohol comes in several forms with a multitude of purposes. While simple alcohols are drying and often irritating, other types are not. In fact, some are emollients that make your skin feel soft and smooth.

Skincare products use three different kinds of alcohols in formulations: simple, fatty, and aromatic.

Simple Alcohols

Thin, clear, and water-like, simple alcohols are commonly used in toners because they dry the skin. Frequent use of products with simple alcohols might cause skin irritation. When people say, "Don't use alcohol," they are referring to simple alcohols. This type of alcohol might be listed as ethyl alcohol (ethanol), isopropyl alcohol, SD alcohol, denatured alcohol, or alcohol on skincare labels.*

Fatty Alcohols

With a more complex chemical structure than simple alcohols, fatty alcohols are typically oily or waxy. Used most commonly as emulsifiers to stabilize a mixture of oil-and-water ingredients, they keep these two types of ingredients from separating. They also have emollient properties that give your skin a smooth velvety feel. They are not drying. Examples include: cetearyl alcohol, caprylic alcohol, stearyl alcohol, cetyl alcohol, and lauryl alcohol.

---

* Denatured or SD alcohol is a term for ethyl alcohol with added poison to make it toxic. Because the government regulates and taxes ethyl alcohol designated for human consumption, what you buy in a bar or liquor store is much more expensive than rubbing alcohol. Denatured or SD Alcohol remains inexpensive for topical use, but it's poisoned so people won't drink it.

Aromatic Alcohols

Oily with a fruity smell, aromatic alcohols can function as a preservative or as a fragrance. Benzyl alcohol is a good example of an aromatic alcohol.

Consumer Demand vs. Effectiveness

Manufacturers spend an inordinate amount of time, energy, and money to develop skincare products that sell. Most major companies use focus groups to find out what is trending and what products consumers would buy. They bring products to market based on these studies. The desires of the consumer population take top priority in skincare product development.

The perfect moisturizer reduces water loss from skin and restores its ability to retain water. It does not cause any allergic reactions, nor does it clog pores. Additionally, it is pleasing to the user, affordable, easily available, and long lasting. The perfect moisturizer provides immediate benefit.

Although excellent moisturizers are available, the perfect moisturizer does not exist. Grandma's recommendation to use 100% white petrolatum, which most people know as Vaseline®, is some of the best advice you'll ever get—if you don't mind the greasy feeling. Moisturizers that aren't as greasy simply aren't as effective at preventing water loss from the skin.

"The perfect moisturizer does not exist."

When people ask me to name the perfect moisturizer, I tell them, "You'll have to find the one that's perfect for you."

My patients express frustration when I say that. They feel unsure because they have no way to determine whether a product is actually good for them. Most people select products because of their experience when using it:

- How it feels.
- Its smell.
- The type of dispenser.
- Whether it meets an immediate need, such as soothing rough skin, calming itchiness, or improving the appearance of their skin.

People with skin conditions such as acne and eczema have more challenges because certain ingredients cause them irritation. That's why I developed the Product Selector on FryFace. com and offer it free to the public. The science available to determine which ingredients trigger conditions like acne and eczema is far from complete, so I always recommend that patients with skin conditions seek medical advice.

I also suggest my patients use moisturizers from reputable companies that have the resources to consistently produce effective, safe, and affordable products that are readily available everywhere. Choose one you like.

Some people love a jar. Others want a pump bottle. Some like a tube to carry in their purse or suitcase, still others prefer a flip top. Dispenser type is important because you might pass up an effective product if you don't like its container. Watch out for fancy containers because the most expensive part of many moisturizers is the packaging.

FryFace Rule #4
The cost of a skincare product is not a measure of its effectiveness.

I advise my patients with healthy skin to purchase thicker petrolatum-based products during the winter as they work better at preventing moisture loss when the air is dry. I also tell them it's best to apply moisturizer after showering when a thin film of water coats the skin. During hot humid summer days, when your skin loses less water, lightweight thinner formulations might be more appropriate.

"Moisturize" your skin. It's good for you.

By the way, fireflies aren't really flies. Peanuts aren't really nuts, and strawberries aren't really berries.

CHAPTER 9

The Real (But Often Overlooked) Fountain of Youth: Sunscreen

When I ask my patients if they wear sunscreen, they usually reply, "Yes, whenever I go to the beach."

I then ask, "How many days a year do you go to the beach?" The most common answer is two to seven days, and I respond, "And what about the other 360 days of the year?"

The most common answers to that question: "I don't get sun," or "I'm never outside."

My office is in a four-floor building. The large parking lot surrounding the building has no trees and provides no shade. Since the building is very busy, oftentimes patients have to park quite a distance from the entrance. When I hear, "I don't get sun," or "I'm never outside," I ask them, "Where did you park today?"

Almost immediately, they smile.

My eyebrows go up. "Oh . . . so you did get sun today?"

A little sheepish. "Only two or three minutes."

"And how are you getting back to your car? Another two or three minutes of sunshine on your unprotected face. Do you go to the supermarket or the post office while you're out? Do you stop at the end of your driveway to pick up your mail and chat with your neighbor for a while? Or maybe you pause to pull a stray weed from beside your mailbox. These small minutes add up."

UV light passing through your car window is additional radiation exposure. If you walk your dog or jog, you rack up a lot of time in the sun. If you're like most people, you get hours and hours of incidental sun exposure each week without realizing it—on your face, ears, back of your hands, and on all other exposed skin. It is no accident that a high percentage of skin cancer occurs in these areas.

Somewhere along the way, dermatologists, the media, and sun-safety educational campaigns failed to convince the majority of Americans about the importance of wearing sunscreen every day.* Sunscreen application should be part of your morning ritual the same as brushing your teeth.

> *"Sunscreen application should be part of your morning ritual."*

---

* PR Newswire, "2019 RealSelf Sun Safety Report: Only 1 in 10 Americans Uses Sunscreen Daily; Men Significantly More Likely Than Women to Reapply Sunscreen and Get Annual Skin Check."

Even on cloudy days, your skin is exposed to UV light as it comes through the clouds. When it's raining, apply sunscreen. If the sun comes out later, you probably won't interrupt what you are doing to apply it, especially if you wear makeup. After you dress in the morning, apply sunscreen to all exposed surfaces, and you'll know you're covered. Make an attempt to reapply it later in the day, even over your makeup. That brilliant ball of light in the center of our universe, commonly portrayed as a happy yellow smiley face, emits harmful radiation every single minute that it's above the horizon.

While most everyone knows sunscreen helps prevent sunburn and decreases the likelihood of skin cancer, most people don't know that sunscreen is, bar none, the most effective over-the-counter product to enhance and improve the appearance and health of your skin.

Sunscreen is in a league of its own. It is the real magic potion, a Fountain of Youth that prevents sunspots, wrinkles, and saggy skin. It is the one skincare product that meets expectations, and scientific research clearly shows its benefits.

Overpromised "age-defying" creams don't compare themselves to sunscreen for one simple reason: they can't compete. As a matter of fact, many "anti-aging" products include sunscreen in their formulations as the basis for their anti-aging claims. It is the closest thing we currently have to a true anti-aging, age-defying product. Not only can it reduce the speed of aging, but sunscreen also helps reverse the skin damage caused by the sun, also known as photoaging.*

Dr. Adele Green studied the benefits of applying sunscreen. She measured the amount of photoaging of skin in adults who randomly applied sunscreen with those who applied it daily for

---

* Randhawa, "Daily Use of a Facial Broad Spectrum Sunscreen Over One-Year Significantly Improves Clinical Evaluation of Photoaging," 1354-1361.

four and a half years. Those who applied sunscreen daily showed no detectable increase in photoaging at the end of the study. In addition, regular sunscreen users had 24 percent less skin aging compared to the group who used sunscreen now and then.*

"Sunscreen can reverse signs of photoaging."

These are scientific conclusions based on quality research. When it comes to skin aging, scientists describe two main causes: time and environmental factors.

Time

The speed of chronological aging varies, determined by genetics. We have no control over the timing of this aging process.

As the years progress, your skin produces fine wrinkles. It becomes thin and transparent. It loses its ability to stretch and maintain its shape. Pinch the back of your hand and see how fast it recoils. With age comes the loss of fat under the skin, and our good friend, gravity, pulls the skin down, causing it to sag.

Most of us start to see these changes in our thirties and forties. If you don't start to see these signs of aging until your fifties or sixties, thank your parents.

Environmental Factors

Time is inevitable, but we can control our environment to a large degree. For example, we can consciously avoid cigarette smoking and sun exposure. The most preventable cause of age-related changes in our skin is ultraviolet light. The sun causes deep wrinkles, freckles, and age spots, leathery and rough-appearing skin, warty-like growths, and more.

---

* Hughes, "Sunscreen and Prevention of Skin Aging."

Sun exposure also speeds up the skin's aging process. Just a few minutes of sun exposure each day over the course of many years can cause significant skin damage.

"Sun exposure speeds up the skin's aging process."

If you want to see how sun exposure has affected your skin to date, compare the skin on your face, chest, or shoulders to the skin on your buttocks or any place generally covered by clothing. If you're a light-skinned woman over forty, you'll likely see a big difference in skin tone and texture between those two areas.

Darker skin has more natural protection, so a darker-skinned woman might not see the effects of photoaging until she's in her fifties. Sun-exposed skin becomes freckled and unevenly pigmented. Skin that's usually covered appears much lighter and more evenly pigmented, although all of that person's skin is the same age.

As part of a comprehensive sun protection program, sunscreen usage is recommended by the American Academy of Dermatology, The Skin Cancer Foundation, Centers for Disease Control and Prevention (CDC), and almost every major dermatologic association around the world. It is the most beneficial skincare product on the market.

"Sunscreen is the most beneficial skincare product on the market."

What Is Sunscreen

When applied to your skin, sunscreen helps prevent the sun's ultraviolet rays from reaching the skin surface. Unlike cosmetics, sunscreen is an over-the-counter drug. The FDA requires sunscreen manufacturers to test their products for safety and efficacy.

"Sunscreen is an over-the-counter drug."

The active ingredients that prevent the sun's rays from reaching the skin's surface are called sunscreen filters. In the US, the FDA has approved only sixteen sunscreen filters. Of those sixteen, only eight are in use today. Europe has thirty approved sunscreen filters.

Each of these filters protects the skin from a certain range of ultraviolet radiation. For this reason, multiple filters called active ingredients often appear in the ingredient listing of any given sunscreen. By using more than one filter, the product protects from a wider range of ultraviolet radiation.

Sunscreen is available in two types: chemical and physical. Both types protect the skin from the sun's UV rays. To prevent the sun's rays from penetrating the skin, chemical sunscreens absorb UV light and release heat via chemical reaction. After going through this reaction process for several hours, the chemical breaks down, so fresh sunscreen must be reapplied.

"Chemical sunscreens protect via a chemical reaction."

Chemical sunscreens are colorless, easy to rub into the skin, and they leave an invisible film. They tend to be more affordable, but they are also more likely to cause an allergic reaction, especially for those with sensitive skin or certain skin conditions like eczema. (More on brands and recommendations for sunscreens in Chapter 10 on page 136.)

In contrast, physical sunscreens create a barrier that blocks the UV rays by causing them to reflect and scatter. All physical sunscreens contain zinc oxide, titanium dioxide, or both. They might leave a white cast on the skin surface, a definite nuisance, especially for darker-skinned individuals. Physical sunscreens are less likely to cause allergic reactions than chemical sunscreens, so we often recommend them for children and individuals with sensitive skin.

"Physical sunscreens create a barrier that blocks the UV rays."

All sunscreens are chemicals. One type absorbs the UV rays and goes through a chemical reaction. The other blocks the rays and reflects them. How they work determines whether they are in the chemical or physical classification.

Selecting a Sunscreen

The sunscreen aisle can be overwhelming. Each package has giant-sized numbers after SPF with the words "broad spectrum" or "stick application." You'll find sunscreen for babies, sports enthusiasts, and beachgoers although no specific sunscreen filter or formulation is unique to any of them. When making a buying decision on sunscreen, here are my recommendations:

Broad Spectrum

Two types of sun rays reach the earth's surface: ultraviolet A (UVA), which are the dominant tanning rays, and ultraviolet B (UVB), the dominant burning rays. Longer UVA rays penetrate deeply into your skin's surface. These rays go through glass windows. Whether exposure comes from outdoor sunlight or tanning parlor salons, UVA rays cause skin damage. Shorter UVB rays cause sunburn and skin cancers. Sunscreens labeled Broad Spectrum protect from both types of ultraviolet rays.

> *"Broad Spectrum sunscreen protects from both the shorter and longer UV rays."*

SPF 30 or Higher

SPF, or Sun Protection Factor, measures the amount of sunburn protection the sunscreen provides. The SPF number shows the amount of solar energy required to cause sunburn while someone wears sunscreen compared to the amount of energy required to cause sunburn on untreated skin.

As the SPF increases, so does sunburn protection. An SPF of 30 prevents 97 percent of the burning rays (UVB) from reaching the skin's surface. An SPF of 50 prevents 98 percent of UVB rays from reaching the surface of your skin. No sunscreen provides 100 percent protection.

With an increase of only 1 percent, are sunscreens with higher than SPF 30 necessary? Yes, studies show sunscreen with higher SPF is better at preventing sunburn.* SPF 100 performed better than SPF 50. Of course, how you use the product will ultimately determine its efficacy. Missed spots or application of too little product provide less than favorable results.

> *"Sunscreen with higher SPF is better at preventing sunburn."*

---

* Williams, "SPF 100+ sunscreen is more protective against sunburn than SPF 50+ in actual use: Results of a randomized, double-blind, split-face, natural sunlight exposure clinical trial," 902-910.e2.

Water resistant

Based on standard testing, sunscreens that maintain their declared SPF protection after forty minutes of water immersion may put *water-resistant* on their label. The FDA no longer allows manufacturers to label sunscreens as waterproof or sweatproof. They can't identify their products as sunblocks either because these claims overstate their effectiveness.

To sum it up, the best sunscreen is broad-spectrum and water-resistant with an SPF of 30 or higher used daily, liberally, and often.

"The best sunscreen is broad-spectrum and water-resistant with an SPF of 30 or higher used daily, liberally, and often."

Spray, lotion, cream, or stick—it doesn't matter. Just find a sunscreen product you like. Sprays are easy to use which make them a favorite type, especially for moms because they can apply them to children running away. Never spray sunscreen directly onto your face. Spray the sunscreen onto your hands, and then apply it to your face. If you worry about sunscreen causing eye burn, select a solid wax-based stick that is less likely to run into your eyes when you exercise and sweat.

As a general rule, an average-sized adult in a bathing suit should apply enough sunscreen to fill a shot glass. It's important to evenly apply enough product over all exposed skin to reach the amount of SPF protection printed on the label. Reapply every two hours if swimming or sweating excessively.

Don't forget that lip balm should contain sunscreen as well. I see far too many patients who have skin cancer on their lip because they forgot to apply lip balm with SPF.

"Don't forget that lip balm should contain sunscreen."

Common Concerns about Sunscreen

To be very clear, the benefits of wearing sunscreen on exposed skin far outweigh the risk of not doing so. As with everything, always consider the benefit-risk ratio of your actions. Here are some news stories recently seen in media:

1. Sunscreen usage causes vitamin D deficiency.

A thorough review of studies on vitamin D and sun exposure over the past fifty years shows little evidence that sunscreen causes vitamin D deficiency when used in real-life conditions. More importantly, no evidence negates current recommendations to wear sunscreen in order to prevent skin cancer.

Yes, adequate vitamin D levels are important for optimal health. With medical guidance, should low vitamin D levels occur, use supplementation if necessary.*

2. Sunscreen ingredients cause hormonal disruption and cancer.

Based on studies where rats were fed high doses of these ingredients, several watchdog groups declared sunscreen filters to be unsafe. They claimed that exposure to these ingredients caused hormonal disruption and cancer.

First of all, no one is suggesting that sunscreen should be eaten. To minimize ingestion, I recommend using lip balms formulated with SPF protection rather than applying regular sunscreen on your lips. To date, no scientific evidence shows that sunscreen is harmful to humans when applied in a reasonable and customary way.

3. Sunscreen ingredients are absorbed into the blood.

In recent studies, laboratory scientists applied commercially available chemical sunscreen to test subjects, under maximal use conditions, covering 75 percent of the body four times a day for several days (rarely done in real-life conditions). When subjects had

---

* Neale, "The effect of sunscreen on vitamin D: a review," 907-915.

their blood tested, several active ingredients from these sunscreens were present at a level where the FDA mandated further safety testing. From these studies, the FDA concluded further studies are warranted to assure the safety of these ingredients. * They also stressed that the study doesn't prove sunscreen ingredients cause harm.

Those who want to play it safe while waiting for further studies should select physical sunscreens containing titanium dioxide or zinc oxide. These ingredients are deemed safe. Most importantly, the study concluded that individuals should *not* refrain from using sunscreen.

> *"The study concluded that individuals should not refrain from using sunscreen."*

4. Sunscreen is killing the coral reefs.

In 2008, Italian scientists placed small fragments of coral and sunscreen in plastic bags for a few days. The coral in the bags became infected with viruses and bleached. The authors concluded "up to 10 percent of the world reefs are potentially threatened by sunscreen-induced coral bleaching." Coral bleaching happens when coral turns white due to the disappearance of algae that usually lives within the coral tissue.

In a 2016 study**, one-day-old coral larvae (not intact coral colonies) were placed in artificial seawater and exposed to various concentrations of the sunscreen filter, oxybenzone. After a

---

* Matta, "Effect of Sunscreen Application Under Maximal Use Conditions on Plasma Concentration of Sunscreen Active Ingredients: A Randomized Clinical Trial," 2082–2091.

** Downs, "Toxicopathological Effects of the Sunscreen UV Filter, Oxybenzone (Benzophenone-3), on Coral Planulae and Cultured Primary Cells and Its Environmental Contamination in Hawaii and the US Virgin Islands."

few hours, the coral larvae became pale (bleached). The authors concluded that oxybenzone threatens the resilience of coral reefs to water temperature changes due to climate change.

When that information reached the media, it caused a wave of concern, and lawmakers in Hawaii banned the sale of sunscreens containing two particular sunscreen filters: oxybenzone and octinoxate. Both studies took place in a laboratory using artificial water. And the amount of sunscreen in the lab far exceeded the amount caused by swimmers and divers around coral reefs in the wild.

Terry Hughes, director of the Australian Research Council Centre of Excellence for Coral Reef Studies at James Cook University, did not agree with these conclusions. Hughes said: "The conclusion from the media is sunscreen is killing the world's coral, and that's laughable . . . Many reefs are remote, without tourists, and many of them nonetheless are showing impact from climate change . . . if you want to study global threats, you have to look on a global scale and they haven't done that."*

Hughes went on to say, "The biggest stresses are climate change, overfishing, and pollution, and pollution more generally than sunscreen," Hughes said. "Sunscreen, because of its source, is far less of a problem than runoff of pesticides in rivers."**

Insufficient evidence links sunscreen use to harming the coral reefs. Don't throw away your oxybenzone-containing sunscreen just yet.

A modern fallacy I see all the time is that many people assume sunscreen gives them full clearance to stay in the glaring sun for hours and hours. For optimum skin health everyone should minimize their sun exposure and reduce the need for sunscreen by taking these steps:

---

* Bogle, "No, your sunscreen isn't killing the world's coral reefs."

** Ibid.

- Seek shade during peak hours.
- Cover your skin with long sleeves, a brimmed hat, and loose fitted pants. Besides sun avoidance, wearing clothing provides the best ultraviolet light protection. Cover up, so you can apply sunscreen to smaller regions of the body.
- Minimize the chance that you ingest any sunscreen filters by using lip balm with SPF instead of rubbing regular sunscreen on the lips.
- At night, use a moisturizer that does not contain sunscreen.
- Keep young children out of the sun. Infants under six months old should not be exposed to sunscreen filters because their skin surface area to body mass ratio is quite high. I advise keeping infants under one year old out of direct sun exposure. They won't complain. I promise. As for older infants and young toddlers, cover them up with protective clothing to limit the amount of skin that needs protection via sunscreen.
- When you must be in direct sunlight, sunscreen is the absolute best choice. Again, the risk of UV exposure without sunscreen far outweighs the risk of using these products.

Frequent Questions

Questions about sunscreen frequently arise in my office. Here are a few I'm asked most often:

Q: Who should wear sunscreen?

A: Everyone. Men, women, and children over six months of age. Grandmothers and grandfathers. Teachers, lawyers, and health-care workers. Individuals with dark complexions and those with lighter complexions. Individuals who burn readily and those who don't. People who tan easily; those who never tan and those who already have a tan. Dog walkers, bicyclers, runners, skiers, gardeners, and beachgoers should wear sunscreen. Apply it daily, liberally, and often.

"Apply sunscreen daily, liberally, and often."

Q: Can I use a moisturizer with SPF instead of applying a second product?

A: My patients often ask me about wearing moisturizers with SPF instead of regular sunscreen. Obtaining the full benefit of any sunscreen product depends on liberal and frequent application. Moisturizers with SPF are rarely applied liberally and almost never reapplied during the day.

The same is true for makeup foundation with SPF. One would have to apply multiple layers of liquid foundation or powder to get the full sun protection factor listed on the product label. Moisturizers and makeup with SPF do provide some protection, so using them is better than using no sun protection at all. However, with customary use a moisturizer-SPF combination rarely provides the SPF protection on the product label. I recommend you use two products: a moisturizer and a separate sunscreen. Many of my patients apply sunscreen in the morning and a moisturizer in the evening when they don't need sunscreen.

"A moisturizer-SPF combination rarely provides the SPF protection on the product label."

Q: Which product should I apply first?

A: For body products, the answer is an easy one. If you need to moisturize, do so after your morning shower. Wait to apply sunscreen until after you get dressed.

As for facial product application, unfortunately, no double-blind studies prove the best way to apply products. Some skin experts recommend you apply moisturizer first and wait until the skin dries before applying sunscreen. Others recommend you put on sunscreen first. Still other experts say to apply a moisturizer first when using a physical sunscreen, but when using a chemical sunscreen, the sunscreen goes on first to create a film on the skin before applying moisturizer.

Before making a complicated decision on this question, ask yourself: Do I need a moisturizer in the morning at all? During warm humid days, I don't apply moisturizer in the morning, only sunscreen. As a matter of fact, on warm humid days I don't need to moisturize my face in the evening either. As the days get longer and drier and the need to moisturize in the morning increases, I apply my moisturizer first, regardless of whether I am using a physical or chemical sunscreen. If I wear makeup that day, I put it on last.

Sunscreen is an ordinary product that most people take for granted. It hangs out in the bottom of their beach bag from September to June with the colorful towels and flip flops—the unsung hero of skin health. Although it doesn't usually come in a pretty little jar and seldom looks pearlescent or sparkly like high-priced lotions, sunscreen is good for you. It is readily available, affordable, safe, and easy to use. The benefits of wearing sunscreen far outweigh the downsides.

Don't forget that sunscreen is regulated as a drug. It can legally claim to change the skin and prevent disease—and it does.

"Sunscreen is a drug. It can legally claim to change the skin and prevent disease—and it does."

Consider the difference in cost between a sunscreen that you can purchase at your local drugstore for $27 per pound and a boutique "anti-aging" cream at $4,734 per pound. Maybe that's another reason why you'd be hard pressed to find a double-blind study comparing the benefits of sunscreen to the benefits of a trendy cosmetic, which legally cannot change the skin.

While I do encourage everyone to use sunscreen, my advice to women is:

Don't use sunscreen because you feel inadequate.

Don't use it because of fine lines around your eyes that you earned or because of a little dark spot on your cheek.

Definitely, don't use it because of wrinkles perfectly placed around your mouth from years of smiling and laughing.

Yes, wearing sunscreen might diminish those badges of honor, but don't wear sunscreen because of them.

Wear sunscreen because it is good for you. In my experience, no other beauty product can compare.

CHAPTER 10

Recommended Products

When I first organized this material for my website, my goal was to deliver an easy-to-understand explanation of how to identify the good guys in skincare vs. the snake-oil salesmen. I know the difference between helpful wording and hype on skincare product labels. I speak the language of ingredient listings. I have the means to test the efficacy of moisturizers and consider their cost and availability. I used this information to create the database on FryFace.com.

However, as I explored all the choices for this book, things got complicated fast. We have effective vs. ineffective products, ethical claims vs. overpromising ones, necessary vs. unnecessary products, not to mention addressing the whole concept of beauty and the difference between a woman's real value vs. celebrity-based ideals and magazine photo fantasies.

I started thinking that the real good guys aren't in high-rise corporate buildings that distribute creams, lotions, and potions to global markets. The real good guys are the people in your life who embrace *you*, the people who *believe you* are fabulous, the people who *know you* are not only enough but you are a treasure.

The celebrity good guys are women like Helen Mirren, Judi Dench, and Sigourney Weaver who embrace themselves as the gorgeous women they are at any age. The good guys are women like Julia Roberts—five-time winner of *People's* Most Beautiful—a fifty-plus woman who tried forehead injections once and said, "Never again" because she valued her own uniqueness. She simply wanted to look like herself.*

> *"Aging is natural and doesn't require a remedy."*

Let's not forget that healthy skin can be mature or youthful. Age is not something to cure because it's not a defect or a disease. So much noise around skincare focuses on aging that the topic often finds its way into my articles and seminars, but the appearance of aging is natural and doesn't require a remedy. Our minds and emotions look for a remedy because of cultural and societal pressures.

Think of it this way. When you glimpse your edgy neighbor heading up your driveway, you might dash to fix your hair and smooth your face before opening the door and flashing her a polite smile. Your blood pressure is a little higher, and your heart rate is too.

When your best friend comes over, a completely different scenario happens. You throw the door open and invite her in. Your bad hair day and lack of makeup is the last thing on your mind.

---

* Brara, "5 Things You Didn't Know About Julia Roberts."

She loves you for who you are, so you feel relaxed and at ease. You're comfortable with who you are. That level of comfort is what I'm talking about.

"No company or brand has a quick fix."

When we go out in public, most of us feel the need to measure up. Cosmetic marketing promises a Magic Wand in a jar or tube, but in reality, no company or brand has a quick fix. Healthy skin comes from a healthy body. This means more than rubbing on a cream or lotion before leaving for work in the morning.

It involves—you guessed it—good food choices and exercise, along with enough sleep, an effective moisturizer, sunscreen, and a healthy dose of fun and laughter. Most ads show photos of healthy, smiling women with glowing skin because health and happiness are major contributors to great skin. What the ads don't tell you: that combination doesn't live inside a pretty little jar.

FryFace Rule #5
The best recipe for healthy, optimal appearing skin is a healthy lifestyle. Magic potions don't exist. If a promise seems too good to be true, it probably is.

Exercise is important for a healthy body. A recent study conducted by McMaster University showed that "Exercise truly is the fountain of youth."* Researchers had subjects go through endurance exercise training three times a week. This group

---

* Tarnopolsky, "Endurance exercise prevents premature aging: McMaster study."

looked significantly younger than their sedentary counterparts.* So, if you want to look and feel younger, go for a walk or run! If you have physical limitations, find a different way to increase your heart rate and work up a sweat. Do it consistently and often. The American Heart Association recommends 150 minutes per week or five thirty-minute workouts a week.**

While staying active, you will also want to avoid the following: smoking, alcohol, sunbathing, and tanning booths. A naive twenty-year-old might think a tan is sexy, but she will pay the price when she's forty. Photoaging is real. The best anti-aging potion is sunscreen.

> *"The best anti-aging potion is sunscreen."*

Reputable Manufacturers

When choosing moisturizer and sunscreen, purchase products from reputable manufacturers. These large companies have a reputation to uphold. Black marks on their record could cause them to lose substantial profits. Smaller manufacturers don't have the resources of their major competitors, so larger companies have an advantage when it comes to:

- Producing consistent products.
- Effectively testing and evaluating their products.
- Distributing their products at the best price point.
- Self-policing, and oftentimes maintaining a membership in good standing with the prestigious Personal Care Products Council.

---

* Ibid.

** American Heart Association, "American Heart Association Recommendations for Physical Activity in Adults and Kids."

The Personal Care Products Council (PCPC) is "the leading national trade association representing the global cosmetics and personal care products industry."* They expect their members to comply with the Consumer Commitment Code to ensure that members provide safe high-quality products.** As a result, cosmetics is one of the safest product categories regulated by the FDA.*** The PCPC offers several valuable services including:

- Links to ingredient buyer guides on their website.
- Online databases.
- Voluntary reporting programs.
- Cosmetic ingredient reviews by independent scientists in bona fide research laboratories.
- Environmentalist chemists conducting toxicology testing for safety both for the user and the environment.

PCPC members include L'Oreal®, Johnson & Johnson® (parent company of Aveeno® and Neutrogena®), and Beiersdorf® (parent company of Eucerin® and Aquaphor®), to name a few. The Personal Care Product Council lists all members on its website.****

Many smaller companies simply don't have the resources for product consistency, testing, global distribution, and PCPC membership. While the lack of these things doesn't necessarily mean that their products are unsafe or less effective, still they cannot provide the validation larger companies can.

Purchasing a product from a company with adequate distribution makes sense. Finding items for your daily skincare

---

* Personal Care Products Council, "Home."

** Personal Care Products Council, "Consumer Commitment Code."

*** Ibid.

**** Personal Care Products Council, "Member Companies."

> *"Purchasing a product from a company with adequate distribution makes sense."*

regimen won't be a problem when you're traveling or moving to a new location.

Sunscreen

I rely on medical journals and independent evaluation from resources like Consumer Reports for information on sunscreen. This product is closely regulated with advance testing and proof for claims, as any drug would be.

All sunscreens are not created equal. Well-formulated chemical sunscreens outperform mineral sunscreens when it comes to efficacy. As a matter of fact, Consumer Reports' 2022 top recommended sunscreens are all chemical sunscreens.* I ask my patients about their experiences with various brands of sunscreen and their main concerns are stickiness, greasiness, leaving a white cast on the skin, and eye burn. (I covered this topic in much more detail in Chapter 9 on page 115.)

Based on thirty years of dermatologic patient experience and consumer-report objective testing, I feel comfortable recommending two of my favorite sunscreens:

- LaRoche-Posay® Anthelios 60 Melt-In Sunscreen Milk (CR high performing)**: lightweight, no white cast, non-greasy.

---

* https://www.consumerreports.org/products/sunscreens-34523/sunscreen -33614/recommended/

** https://www.laroche-posay.us/sunscreen/anthelios-melt-in-sunscreen- milk-spf-60-883140500322.html?GeoRedirectOff&gclid=Cj0KCQiA2ITu BRDkARIsAMK9Q7M8Og6GREKjo2xlZDD1x8hePLGmlhtqxtHuZJ_8 4fJauilh9if5QYAaAg4YEALw_wcB

- Banana Boat Sport Ultra Sunscreen Stick SPF 50+*: non-sticky, no white cast.

  Because this product is wax based, it's less likely to run into the eyes and cause burning when users sweat excessively due to intense heat or exercise. As an added bonus, you'll never have to touch the product, as it is applied much like a deodorant stick, directly onto the skin.

My Own Testing

I want to recommend products that are not only cosmetically pleasing but also truly effective, so I began my own testing process back in 2015. As a result of my research experience and science training, I knew that research laboratory testing involves control groups, double blind studies, closely regulated conditions, and hundreds of comparison samples repeated hundreds of times. My office is a busy dermatology practice. No way would I have time to run a research facility as well.

So, I took a different approach. I tested the practical application of moisturizers on patients in the course of their normal daily lives. All of my test subjects were volunteers, mostly patients, but some family and friends also donated their time. Some volunteers chose to test their favorite moisturizer to compare its effectiveness against other products. I offered some volunteers two different moisturizers of my own choosing.

All of the test subjects had healthy skin without any inflammatory skin condition such as eczema, acne, or psoriasis. The patient-volunteers were in my office for an unrelated issue, such as removing a mole or a wart.

---

* https://www.bananaboat.com/products/banana-boat-sport-ultra -sunscreen-stick-spf-50

My sampling of volunteers came from all age groups. I tested fifteen-year-olds through seventy-year-olds. The majority were women between forty and sixty-five, of all skin types and ethnicities. In a research laboratory, these variations would be segmented into individual studies. I focused on simply measuring skin hydration to find trends, rather than detailed statistics. In this practical study, my goal was to determine which products effectively and consistently raised skin hydration levels.

Before beginning a moisturizer comparison test, I took a measurement to determine the baseline hydration on the most superficial layer of forearm skin on each volunteer. I used the Courage & Khazaka Corneometer® CM 825*, the same instrument used by NASA to determine the state of the skin of astronauts on board the International Space Station (ISS). This machine gives exact, reproducible measurements.

I gave my volunteers specific instructions:

1. Discontinue using any moisturizer or body oil for at least one week before beginning their test.
2. Continue their usual washing routine with their own soap or cleanser during the test.
3. Apply a dime-sized dollop of each product, one on the left forearm, the other on the right forearm, in the morning after their shower and again at night.
4. Return to the office in one week to retest on the Corneometer®.
5. I asked the question, "Which of these do you like better, and why?" to get a picture of the user experience for each product.

---

* Courage+Khazaka Electronics, "Corneometer CM 825: The World's Most Popular Skin Hydration Measurement Instrument."

I made over one hundred product comparisons, and my research continues to this day. In New York, I don't test during June, July, and August. In high humidity, skin takes moisture from the air, so New York's summer humidity hinders accurate readings.

Although my testing methods do not meet the gold-standard double-blinded placebo-controlled studies of medical science, after completing over one hundred product comparison tests of some of the most common moisturizers on the market, I have a strong sense of which products are effective moisturizers and which are not.

Products that I recommend consistently show increased skin hydration at an acceptable level. When a product consistently tests effectively, I personally test it to validate the findings. Along with consistent hydration, my preferred products also provide a tolerable user experience. Some people are willing to deal with tackiness if the product hydrates the skin. Others don't want any tackiness at all.

The user experiencee also takes into account the smell, thickness, and silkiness of the product. If a user doesn't like the feel of a product, they won't use it. Some people want a smooth and silky feel. Some want a thicker feel. Some prefer a pump bottle over a jar, Some love fragrance, and some are sensitive to fragrance. Each person's preferences are very specific.

At the crossroads where effectiveness meets a pleasant user experience stands the crux of the matter.

> *"Recommended products consistently showed both substantial hydration and an acceptable user experience."*

The product selector at FryFace.com lists more than one hundred products. In the initial survey, you select your personal preferences, such as fragrance-free or oil-free. By clicking acne-prone or eczema-prone, you opt for products without ingredients that aggravate acne or eczema. The software then creates a list of products that fit your criteria.

To keep this simple, I'm releasing my findings for three of my most recommended products (in no particular order) as examples of effective brands that are readily available and affordable. I divided my study into two categories: body moisturizers and face moisturizers. Some products can be used for both.

A Word about Petroleum Jelly

As I briefly mentioned in Chapter 5 on page 76, petroleum jelly is a prime example of an overlooked and undervalued staple in the skincare industry. It is one of the safest and most versatile products on the market. Although produced in pharmaceutical-grade facilities, cosmetic petroleum jelly received a lot of unwarranted bad press tying it to the industrial oil industry. This is an incident of someone striving to gain market share by disparaging a standard product that has been on the market since 1872.*

The fact that petroleum jelly is derived from a waxy material formed on oil rigs scares people. However, these unprocessed waxes are distilled and refined to become pure cosmetic grade petroleum jelly, also called petrolatum USP (United States Pharmacopeia). Petroleum jelly is a refined and purified product that meets the requirements of the United States Pharmacopeia for food, drug, or medicinal use.

> *"Petroleum jelly is the purest, non-comedogenic, non-allergenic product found on skincare aisles."*

---

* Wikipedia contributors, "Vaseline."

Sometimes known as white petrolatum, it is the most effective, non-comedogenic, non-allergenic moisturizing product found on skincare aisles. When other products go through laboratory testing for allergic reactions, petrolatum is the standard negative control because allergic reactions to it are almost unheard of.

Additionally, it reduces water loss through the skin by 98 percent, creating a friendly environment for healing.* An occlusive in skincare formulations, petroleum jelly is an ingredient in more than half of all skincare products sold today, some say up to 75 percent.

> *"Petrolatum is an ingredient in more than half of all skincare products sold today."*

Due to its lubricating and coating properties, petroleum jelly can be used to:

- Soothe dry, cracked skin on problematic areas like elbows and knees.
- Soften dry, cracked heels.
- Heal chapped lips.
- Calm inflamed eyelids.
- Protect skin around the nose when chafed from wind or from overblowing the nose due to a cold.
- Help earring insertion by applying to earring posts.
- Prevent windburn on cheeks.
- Improve nail health by rubbing onto nails and around nail cuticles.
- Tame runaway eyebrows.

---

* Sethi, "Moisturizers: The Slippery Road."

- Assist in hair grooming.
- Prevent inflammation in areas that might chafe during exercise for cyclists, wrestlers, runners, and other athletes.
- Enhance wound repair when applied to superficial cuts and lacerations.
- Treat diaper rash.

It is available everywhere, and it's extremely affordable. A jar of petroleum jelly should be in everyone's bathroom.

Body Moisturizers

1. Eucerin® Advanced Repair Lotion*: consistently high performing and cosmetically pleasing to most users. A few described the product as feeling a little thicker, but that feeling subsided with time.
2. Neutrogena® HydroBoost Body Gel Cream Fragrance-Free**: users consistently described their skin as silky smooth and light after applying this product.
3. Vaseline® Intensive Care™ Advanced Repair Unscented Lotion***: deeply moisturizing for very dry skin. Effective and cosmetically pleasing for most users.

---

* https://www.eucerinus.com/products/repair/eucerin-smoothing-repair-dry-skin-lotion

** https://www.neutrogena.com/skin/neutrogena-hydro-boost-body-gel-cream---fragrance-free/6811344.html

*** https://www.vaseline.com/us/en/products/lotions-and-moisturizers/vaseline-intensive-care-advanced-repair-unscented-lotion.html

Facial Moisturizers

1. CeraVe® PM Facial Moisturizing Lotion*: a lightweight lotion that spreads easily. It contains no sunscreen.
2. La Roche-Posay® Toleriane Double Repair Moisturizer UV Broad Spectrum SPF 30**: a lightweight lotion that leaves a silky feel. It contains a broad-spectrum sunscreen.
3. Olay® Regenerist Micro-Sculpting Cream, Fragrance-free***: this moisturizer comes in a jar. It spreads instantly on the skin. Users love the feel of this product. It does not contain sunscreen.

Lip Balm

Lip balm is a skincare product that is both a protectant and a moisturizer. The skin on your lips is very thin and has few sweat glands. They are susceptible to sun damage, so lip balm with sunscreen is an important product.

Testing lips with the Corneometer® isn't practical since lip balm is washed off regularly with food and drink, and we constantly moisten our lips with saliva. With my limited scope, I didn't attempt testing. I base my recommendation on the ingredient list.

Some people don't like the burning feeling caused by camphor and menthol. Some want flavors and they like a waxy feel. Lip balm preferences are very subjective.

---

* https://www.cerave.com/skincare/moisturizers/pm-facial-moisturizing-lotion

** https://www.laroche-posay.us/face-and-body-skin-care/face-products/face-moisturizer/toleriane-double-repair-facial-moisturizer-with-spf-3337875545846.html

*** https://www.olay.com/en-us/skin-care-products/regenerist-micro-sculpting-cream-fragrance-free-moisturizer

1. ChapStick® Classic Original lip protectant* is still my favorite. It does contain camphor, but it does not contain menthol, a common cause of burn.
2. Vaseline® Lip Therapy® Advanced Healing** (in a tube) and Original*** (in a jar) is a petroleum jelly product. Great for inside winter application or for chapped lips from the sniffles.
3. Aquaphor® Lip Repair**** contains shea butter and beeswax for long-lasting protection. It's also available with sunscreen, SPF 30.*****
4. Blistex® Five Star Lip Protection******: formulated to protect the lips from the harshest conditions and contains broad spectrum sunscreen, SPF 30.

Unnecessary Products

Without mentioning any particular brand, I'd like to address a few products that consistently lose in the comparison study of my in-office testing. Three examples of poorly performing moisturizers are:

1. Organic creams: *Organic* is a marketing term that tells you this product contains plant extracts and oils. An

---

* https://www.chapstick.com/category/chapstick-classic/products/classic/original

** https://www.vaseline.com/us/en/products/lip-care/vaseline-lip-therapy-advanced-healing-tube.html?bvstate=pg:2/ct:r

*** https://www.vaseline.com/us/en/products/lip-care/vaseline-lip-therapy-original-mini.html

**** https://www.aquaphorus.com/aquaphor-lip-repair/

***** https://www.aquaphorus.com/aquaphor-lip-protectant-sunscreen/

****** https://www.blistex.com/products/five-star-lip-protection/

overwhelming majority of organic creams fare poorly in Corneometer® testing. They often have an unpleasant smell, an oily feel and, like any plant-based oil, they can be allergens. Creams containing petroleum jelly and silicone derivatives perform much better than these do, with less potential for irritation and fewer allergens.

2. Coconut oil: Those looking for a plant-based moisturizer often use coconut oil. I tested coconut oil against a large number of products with the same results every time. Coconut oil consistently fails to provide an environment that yields adequately hydrated skin. By itself, coconut oil makes your skin feel soft and smooth, but it doesn't prevent your skin from losing water. It is a poor moisturizer and doesn't reach the minimum level for adequate hydration on the Corneometer® test.

3. Direct sales skincare lines: Many direct sales products do not perform well in Corneometer® testing yet can cost up to $2,500 per pound. Although this seems like a sweeping generalization, I have yet to find one that performs well enough to merit the cost. But I'm still looking!

Based on my test results, I feel confident steering my patients toward products that are genuinely beneficial because I have numbers to back up my recommendations.

A Skincare Routine for Healthy Skin

An effective skincare regimen can be both easy and affordable. I put together a suggested routine. Of course, this is adaptable to individual preferences. The following regimen is for healthy skin. Individuals with acne, rosacea, eczema, or other skin conditions should consult their dermatologist for daily skincare recommendations.

In the Morning

1. *Cleanse* your face with warm water. This can be done during your morning shower. In my unpublished study of over five hundred women with healthy skin, more than half of them preferred cleansing with water alone. I include myself in this group. Women with oily skin might prefer a mild cleansing beauty bar or lipid-free cleanser.

2. *Moisturize* your face if your skin is dry, using an effective product that feels good to you. Some women do not need to moisturize every morning. During the cold winter months when the air is dry, the need to moisturize increases. During hot and humid summer days, moisturizing might be less necessary. In cold dry climates, don't forget to moisturize the body after every shower.

3. Apply *sunscreen* with SPF 30 or higher to your face, neck, hands, and all exposed skin every single day, 365 days a year. Broad-spectrum sunscreens offer longer-lasting protection than moisturizers that contain SPF. The sunscreen in moisturizers is rarely water resistant. And all too often, it doesn't last as long.

I recommend you use a broad-spectrum sunscreen after applying moisturizer each morning, if you choose to use a moisturizer. If time or money is an issue, using a moisturizer with SPF is better than nothing. Remember: apply sunscreen liberally to achieve the SPF listed on the product label.

If you work outdoors, apply a water-resistant sunscreen with SPF 30 or higher to all sun-exposed areas. Reapply every two hours when activity or sweating could cause the product to wash off.

In the Evening

1. *Cleanse* your face with warm water. If you prefer, use a mild cleanser to help remove make-up and sebum from oil glands.
2. *Moisturize* your face. Again, the need to moisturize will vary based on the season and the needs of your individual skin. Apply a body moisturizer if the skin is dry, especially in cold dry climates.

Along with an effective skincare regimen, always keep FryFace Rule #6 in mind:

FryFace Rule #6
You are fabulous the way you are. When in doubt, look in the mirror and repeat, "Dear Me, I'm Awesome!"

CHAPTER 11

Beautiful You

Why do accomplished, intelligent women spend so much money on skincare products that don't work?

Maybe because it's fun. Walking away from the makeup counter carrying pretty packages filled with gleaming jars and skincare samples has its own kind of rush. Fun is good.

Perhaps we buy so many unnecessary products because we like the way our skin feels when we use them. Maybe it's the alluring fragrance. Purchasing a product because it creates an enjoyable experience is okay. Women should pamper themselves, and feel beautiful while they do it.

Unfortunately, my experience as a skin expert tells me that, all too often, the answer to the question, "Why?" has nothing to do with fun or aesthetic pleasures.

For more than thirty years in my dermatology practice, I've experienced the pain and humiliation of thousands of women— and some men—who believe they are inadequate. They invest a lot of time, money, and emotional equity on cosmetics that scientifically cannot possibly do what they promise.

They buy because they feel compelled to fix something they perceive as flawed.

Why? We've been brainwashed.

From the very moment we are born, we absorb the notion that our self-worth is wrapped up in the size of our waistlines, the shape of our noses, and the clarity of our skin. This emphasis on our physical attributes becomes deeply instilled over the years, reinforced by thousands of intentional and subliminal messages on a daily basis—complements of magazine beauty ads, television commercials, and online marketing campaigns in our celebrity-obsessed culture.

If the beauty industry stopped objectifying us, it would cease to exist. What could they sell if we accepted ourselves as we are, superficial imperfections and all?

> *"If the beauty industry stopped objectifying us, it would cease to exist."*

The ads tell us our skin must be flawless with a healthy glow and, above all, we must look youthful. Hence, the barrage of anti-aging, anti-wrinkle, firming, and toning creams that fly off the shelves in a $25.9 billion market.*

We see ads filled with mixed messages like this one, "Feel confident in your own skin and reduce the appearance of your fine lines." If they really want us to feel confident, the ad would read, "Love yourself, even with your fine lines."

---

* "Anti-aging Services Market Size, Share & Trends Analysis Report By Demographics, By Type (Chemical Peel, BOTOX, Microdermabrasion, Breast Augmentation, Liposuction), And Segment Forecasts, 2019 – 2026."

Look closely at product labels and you will see terms like *rejuvenating* and *renewal* plastered all over them. In subtle and not-so-subtle ways, most of society bought into the message that beauty means youthful. This is an unobtainable, unrealistic ideal based purely on cultural norms. All physical beauty fades with time.

Why are we so obsessed with forehead wrinkles, or with any wrinkle for that matter? When and why did the natural aging process become such an exhausting, costly battle?

> *"When and why did the natural aging process become such an exhausting, costly battle?"*

Aging has many benefits that we rarely hear about. Older people are happier, less angry, and they feel fewer stressors than younger people.* Experience gives them a broader perspective and broader coping skills than younger generations. They find conflicts easier to understand because they see life from different points of view. They come up with resolutions and suggest better compromises than their younger counterparts.** Older individuals are more compassionate. They are wiser.

I applaud the skincare industry for producing some of the safest products on the planet. Well-formulated moisturizers and sunscreen products from reputable manufacturers truly support healthy skin, and I highly recommend them to my patients.

However, I object to a culture so focused on appearance that we can't help but see ourselves as inadequate. I object to an industry that takes advantage of our vulnerable feelings.

---

* Fields, "What's So Good About Growing Old?"

** Grossmann, "Reasoning about social conflicts improves into old age," 107 (16) 7246-7250.

"I object to an industry that takes advantage of our vulnerable feelings."

I encounter these feelings of inadequacy every single day in my office. When I enter the examining room and see a frowning woman with worry in her eyes, after the usual pleasantries I ask, "What brought you in today?"

She points to her face and says, "I have this crease on my forehead."

I inspect the area of concern and continue my examination for suspicious moles and other health-related problems. While I look, I ask, "Why are you so hard on yourself? Do you consider yourself a giving person?"

A suggestion of a smile appears on her face as she nods.

"Are you forgiving?" Another nod. This time her brows rise.

"Are you compassionate?"

"Of course," she says, her voice firm.

"Are you kind?" More nods.

"Have you ever cared for a sick family member, a friend, or a neighbor when they were in need?"

"Absolutely."

"You sound like a really beautiful person to me. Why are you so worried about this little mark?"

More often than not, her perspective changes. She smiles, and I feel the worry leave her, at least for the moment. I never really know whether these conversations have a long-term positive impact, but I hope and pray that, somehow, she will see herself as a beautiful person for more than a fleeting moment. I hope she likes herself for who she is rather than dwelling on her perceived flaws.

"I hope she likes herself for who she is rather than dwelling on her perceived flaws."

Life is not a dress rehearsal. We get one shot at it. Let go of insecurities that keep us down. Stop listening to outside influences that make us feel inadequate, especially those that pull at our heartstrings just to make a sale. Live each day to its fullest.

The skin color we were born with is our perfect skin color. The curl or wave in our hair (or lack thereof) is our perfect head of hair. Who determines if we have too much hair growing on our arms? So what, if we grow hairs in "inappropriate" places? Who sets these standards anyway? So what, if some spots on our skin are darker and other spots are lighter? Big deal.

Do we really want to spend time worrying about something so trivial? Do we really want to spend our hard-earned cash on products that, by law, can't change the skin?

Before purchasing a product, ask yourself, "Am I buying this cosmetic because I want it or because of someone else? Do I really care if my forehead has a fine line or if the area around my eyes creases a bit when I smile?"

Instead, let's celebrate our triumphs and surround ourselves with supportive people who value us for who we are. Kindness matters. Health matters. Accomplishments matter. None of those things come in a tube or bottle.

When you get down on yourself, and even when you're not, take a moment to look into the mirror. Give yourself a big smile and say those four little words, "Dear Me, I'm Awesome."

Because, my friend, you truly are.

At FryFace.com, We Believe

You are fabulous. All too often, the marketing for skincare products sends the message that you are inadequate, that you need to look different, that you need to look younger, that your appearance is flawed. We believe you are perfect the way you are, and so should you.

Choose a simple skincare regimen with products that benefit your skin health based on valid science. Many skincare products have no proven benefit and may even be harmful to your skin. All you need for optimal skin health is a well-formulated moisturizer and sunscreen.

Safe, effective, and affordable skincare products are readily available at local pharmacies and drugstores. You do not need to spend a lot of money to optimize your skin health and appearance. The cost of a skincare product is not a measure of its effectiveness.

FryFace.com is not affiliated with any skincare brands, nor are we paid to promote or include any products on our site. FryFace.com is a free service to help you find products that meet your specific needs.

The FryFace Rules

Over the years, I've found myself repeating certain statements again and again. Eventually, I made a list of the ones I say the most, both in speaking and in print. I call them the FryFace Rules. This simple list provides some general guidelines for when you're standing at that beauty wall in the pharmacy or big-box store.

Rule #1
Science has yet to discover a single product or ingredient that can reverse the aging process.

Rule #2
The most important information on a skincare bottle is the ingredient listing.

Rule #3
By law, over-the-counter cosmetics, including facial moisturizers, cannot intend to change the structure or function of skin or they'd be classified as drugs.

Rule #4
The cost of a skincare product is not a measure of its effectiveness.

Rule #5
The best recipe for healthy, optimal appearing skin is a healthy lifestyle. Magic potions don't exist. If a promise seems too good to be true, it probably is.

Rule #6
You are fabulous the way you are. When in doubt, look in the mirror and repeat, "Dear Me, I'm Awesome!"

Bibliography

Ademola, Adedeji. *The real reason why the Himba people Namibia don't bathe.* Face2Face Africa. (Feb. 26, 2018). https://face2faceafrica.com/article/real-reason-himba-people-namibia-dont-bath

Al-Niaimi, Firas, and Nicole Yi Zhen Chiang. *Topical Vitamin C and the Skin: Mechanisms of Action and Clinical Applications.* The Journal of clinical and aesthetic dermatology vol. 10,7 (2017): 14-17.

American Federation of Aging Research. *The Theories of Aging.* Biology of Aging: (NY, NY 2016): 1-9. https://www.afar.org/imported/AFAR_INFOAGING_GUIDE_THEORIES_OF_AGING_2016.pdf

American Heart Association. "American Heart Association Recommendations for Physical Activity in Adults and Kid." *Fitness Basics.* (April 18, 2018). https://www.heart.org/en/healthy-living/fitness/fitness-basics/aha-recs-for-physical-activity-in-adults

"Anti-aging Services Market Size, Share & Trends Analysis Report By Demographics, By Type (Chemical Peel, BOTOX, Microdermabrasion, Breast Augmentation, Liposuction), And Segment Forecasts, 2019–2026" Grandview Research.com. (Feb. 2019). https://www.grandviewresearch.com/industry-analysis/anti-aging-market#:~:text=The%20global%20anti%2Daging%20services%20market%20size%20was%20

estimated%20at,USD%2025.9%20billion%20in%202020.&text=The
%20global%20anti%2Daging%20services%20market%20is%20
expected%20to%20grow,USD%2035.4%20billion%20by%202026

Bennett, Colette. "The best Korean essences to add to your skincare routine."
Daily Dot Bazaar. (Aug. 28, 2018). https://www.dailydot.com/bazaar/
korean-essence/

Berkeley Wellness. *Is Petroleum Jelly Safe?* University of California. (Nov. 24,
2016). https://www.berkeleywellness.com/self-care/over-counter-products
/article/petroleum-jelly-safe

Biron, Bethany. "Beauty has blown up to be a $532 billion industry
—and analysts say that these 4 trends will make it even bigger."
Business Insider. (July 9, 2019). https://www.businessinsider.com/
beauty-multibillion-industry-trends-future-2019-7

Bogle, Ariel. "No, your sunscreen isn't killing the world's coral reefs."
Mashable.com. (Nov. 10, 2015). https://mashable.com/2015/11/10/
sunscreen-killing-coral-reefs/

Brara, Noor. "5 Things You Didn't Know About Julia Roberts." *Vogue
Magazine.* (April 22, 2017). https://www.vogue.com/article/julia-roberts
-5-things-you-didnt-know

Brown, Rita Mae. *Life is too short to be miserable.* Rita Mae Brown Quotes:
BrainyQuote.com, BrainyMedia Inc, 2020. https://www.brainyquote.
com/quotes/rita_mae_brown_454911

Byrd, A., Belkaid, Y. & Segre, J. "The human skin microbiome." *Nat Rev
Microbiol* 16: 143–155 (2018). https://doi.org/10.1038/nrmicro.2017.15

CDC. *Keeping Your hands Clean.* Water, Sanitation, and Environment-
related hygiene. CDC.gov. (Dec. 4, 2019). https://www.cdc.gov/healthy
water/hygiene/hand/handwashing.html

Centers for Disease Control and Prevention. "Burden of Foodborne
Illnesses: Findings." *CDC.* (Nov. 5, 2018) https://www.cdc.gov/food
borneburden/2011-foodborne-estimates.html

Choi, J. M, Lew, V. K., Kimball , A. B. *A single-blinded, randomized, controlled
clinical trial evaluating the effect of face washing on acne vulgaris.* Pediatric
Dermatology, 2006;23(5):421-427. doi:10.1111/j.1525-1470.2006.00276.x

CIR. *Amended Safety Assessment of Parabens as Used in Cosmetics.* Report Data Sheet. (June 19, 2019). https://www.cir-safety.org/sites/default/files/parabe062019TR.pdf

Consumer Reports. Recommended Sunscreens (2022). https://www.consumerreports.org/products/sunscreens-34523/sunscreen-33614/recommended/

Cosmeticsinfo.org. https://cosmeticsinfo.org/ingredient/phenoxyethanol-0 (Under Safety tab)

Courage + Khazaka Electronic GmbH. "Corneometer® CM 825: The World's Most Popular Skin Hydration Measurement Instrument." *C+K electronic.* https://www.courage-khazaka.de/en/16-wissenschaftliche-produkte/alle-produkte/183-corneometer-e

Darbre, P. D., et al. "Concentrations of parabens in human breast tumours." *Journal of applied toxicology : JAT* vol. 24,1 (2004): 5-13. doi:10.1002/jat.958

Davret, Barry. "How To Create Pain And Sell More." *Medium.* (Aug. 23, 2018). https://medium.com/writtenpersuasion/the-art-of-creating-pain-941002a6299c

Dictionary.com, s.v. "Fad (*n.*)." https://www.dictionary.com/browse/fad?s=t

Downs, C. A., Kramarsky-Winter, E., Segal, R. et al. "Toxicopathological Effects of the Sunscreen UV Filter, Oxybenzone (Benzophenone-3), on Coral Planulae and Cultured Primary Cells and Its Environmental Contamination in Hawaii and the US Virgin Islands." *Arch Environ Contam Toxicol* 70, 265–288 (2016). https://doi.org/10.1007/s00244-015-0227-7

Euromonitor Research. *Survey Shows Regional Differences in Bathing Habits Around the World.* Euromonitor International. (July 4, 2014). https://blog.euromonitor.com/survey-shows-regional-differences-in-bathing-habits-around-the-world/

EWG. *EWG Skin Deep.* Cosmetic Database. (2004). https://www.ewg.org/skindeep/

FDA: US Food & Drug Administration. "Are all 'personal care products' regulated as cosmetics?." *FDA.* (Feb. 1, 2016). https://www.fda.gov/industry/fda-basics-industry/are-all-personal-care-products-regulated-cosmetics

FDA: US Food & Drug Administration. *Avage and Tazorac Labeling.* Product. (Nov. 17, 2017). https://www.accessdata.fda.gov/drugsatfda_docs/label/2017/021184s009lbl.pdf

FDA: US Food & Drug Administration. *Cosmetics Compliance & Enforcement.* Cosmetics. (Nov. 3, 2017). https://www.fda.gov/cosmetics/cosmetics-compliance-enforcement

FDA: US Food & Drug Administration. *Cosmetics Labeling Guide.* 21 CFR 701.3(a), (d), (f) (2), (f) (3). Cosmetics. (Nov. 5, 2017). https://www.fda.gov/cosmetics/cosmetics-labeling-regulations/cosmetics-labeling-guide#clgl3

FDA: US Food & Drug Administration. *FDA Authority Over Cosmetics: How Cosmetics Are Not FDA-Approved, but Are FDA-Regulated.* Cosmetics. (Jul. 24, 2018). https://www.fda.gov/cosmetics/cosmetics-laws-regulations/fda-authority-over-cosmetics-how-cosmetics-are-not-fda-approved-are-fda-regulated

FDA: US Food & Drug Administration. *Fragrances in Cosmetics.* Cosmetics. (Aug. 8, 2018). https://www.fda.gov/cosmetics/cosmetic-ingredients/fragrances-cosmetics

FDA: US Food & Drug Administration. *Frequently Asked Questions on Soap.* Cosmetics. (Nov. 11, 2017). https://www.fda.gov/cosmetics/cosmetic-products/frequently-asked-questions-soap

FDA: US Food & Drug Administration. "Is it a Cosmetics, a Drug, or Both? (Or Is It Soap?)." *FDA.* (Aug. 2, 2018). https://www.fda.gov/cosmetics/cosmetics-laws-regulations/it-cosmetic-drug-or-both-or-it-soap#Definedrug

FDA: US Food & Drug Administration. "OTC Drug Facts Label." *FDA.* (Jun. 5, 2015). https://www.fda.gov/drugs/drug-information-consumers/otc-drug-facts-label

FDA: US Food & Drug Administration. *RENOVA (TRETINOIN CREAM 0.02%).* Label. https://www.accessdata.fda.gov/drugsatfda_docs/label/2014/021108s015lbl.pdf

FDA: US Food & Drug Administration. "Wrinkle Treatments and Other Anti-aging Products." *FDA* (Feb. 22, 2018). https://www.fda.gov/cosmetics/cosmetic-products/wrinkle-treatments-and-other-anti-aging-products

FECYT - Spanish Foundation for Science and Technology. "Do we buy cosmetics because they are useful or because they make us feel good?" ScienceDaily.com. http://www.sciencedaily.com/releases/2011/07/110721095846.htm

Federal Trade Commissions. *Fair Packaging and Labeling Act: Regulations Under Section 4 of the Fair Packaging and Labeling Act: 16 C.F.R. 500.* https://www.ftc.gov/enforcement/rules/rulemaking-regulatory-reform-proceedings/fair-packaging-labeling-act-regulations-0

Fields, Helen. "What's So Good About Growing Old?" Smithsonian Magazine. (July 2012). https://www.smithsonianmag.com/science-nature/what-is-so-good-about-growing-old-130839848/

Golden, Robert & Gandy, Jay. *Comment on the publication by Darbre et al.* (2004). Journal of applied toxicology: JAT. 24. 297-9; author reply 299. 10.1002/jat.985.

Goossens, An. *Contact-allergic reactions to cosmetics.* Journal of Allergy vol. 2011 (2011): 467071. doi:10.1155/2011/467071

Grossmann, Igor, et.al., "Reasoning about social conflicts improves into old age." *Proceedings of the National Academy of Sciences* (April 2010): 107 (16) 7246-7250; DOI: 10.1073 /pnas.1001715107

HairStory. "The History of Shampoo." *Essay* (May 19th). https://www.hairstory.com/stories/2017/3/24/the-history-of-shampoo/

Halpern, Allan C., et al. "The Melanoma Letter." *Skin Cancer Foundation: for Medical Providers.* https://provider.skincancer.org/the-melanoma-letter/

Henrich, U, et al. "Experiment Record N° 9392: Skin B." *Erasmus Experiment Archive.* Germany and Slovenia. http://eea.spaceflight.esa.int/portal/exp/?id=9392

Hughes, Maria, et al. "Sunscreen and Prevention of Skin Aging." *Annals of Internal Medicine.* (June 4, 2013). https://doi.org/10.7326/0003-4819-158-11-201306040-00002

Iizuka, H. "Epidermal turnover time." *Journal of dermatological science* vol. 8,3 (1994): 215-7. doi:10.1016/0923-1811(94)90057-4

Insurance Information Institute. *Facts + Statistics: Highway safety.* Auto. https://www.iii.org/fact-statistic/facts-statistics-highway-safety

JAMA Network. "How Many Adverse Events Are Reported to FDA for Cosmetics, Personal Care?" *Post-Embargo News Releases.* (Jun. 26, 2017). https://media.jamanetwork.com/news-item/many-adverse-events-reported -fda-cosmetics-personal-care/

Jones, Oliver and Selinger, Ben. "The chemistry of cosmetics." *Australia Academy of Science.* https://www.science.org.au/curious/people-medicine/ chemistry-cosmetics

Ketchum, Dan. "The Persuasion Technique of Beauty Product Advertising." *Chron.* https://smallbusiness.chron.com/persuasion-techniques-beauty-product-advertising-22993.html

Khanna, Neena, and Siddhartha Datta Gupta. "Rejuvenating facial massage—a bane or boon?." *International journal of dermatology* vol. 41,7 (2002): 407-10. doi:10.1046/j.1365-4362.2002.01511.x

Lee, Michele. *Allure Magazine Will No Longer Use the Term "Anti-Aging."* (Aug. 14, 2017) Issue: *Allure* Magazine Sept. 2017. https://www.allure. com/story/allure-magazine-phasing-out-the-word-anti-aging

Lohrey, Jackie. "Advertising Theories of Cosmetics." *Chron.* https://small business.chron.com/advertising-theories-cosmetics-80185.html

Mae, V. "From Victoria Beckham To Tom Cruise, From The Birdcage To Your Face: The Nightingale Poop Anti-Aging Facial." *Be Youthful.* (Feb. 4, 2013). https://beyouthful.net/from-victoria-beckham-to-tom-cruise-from-the-birdcage-to-your-face-the-nightingale-poop-anti-aging-facial/

Maeda, Kazuhisa. *New Method of Measurement of Epidermal Turnover in Humans.* Cosmetics. Cosmetics (September 24, 2017) 4(4), 47; https:// doi.org/10.3390/cosmetics4040047

Matta MK, Zusterzeel R, Pilli NR, et al. "Effect of Sunscreen Application Under Maximal Use Conditions on Plasma Concentration of Sunscreen Active Ingredients: A Randomized Clinical Trial." *JAMA.* 2019;321(21):2082–2091. doi:10.1001/jama.2019.5586

Nandi, Synjini. *The Fascinating History of Face Masks from Around the World*. Beauty Blog. (Feb. 5, 2019) https://www.nykaa.com/beauty-blog/the-fascinating-history-of-face-masks-from-around-the-world/

National Cancer Institute: Division of Cancer Epidemiology and Genetics. *Alpha-Tocopherol, Beta-Carotene Cancer Prevention (ATBC) Study*. Usa. gov https://atbcstudy.cancer.gov/

Neale, R. E., et al. "The effect of sunscreen on vitamin D: a review." *Br J Dermatol*. 2019 Nov;181(5):907-915. doi: 10.1111/bjd.17980. Epub 2019 Jul 9. PMID: 30945275.

Pererva, Natalia. "The Reasonableness of Rhetorical Questions in Advertisements." *Scripties*. https://scripties.uba.uva.nl/document/168822

Personal Care Products Council. "Consumer Commitment Code." *Questions and Answers*. https://www.personalcarecouncil.org/science-safety/consumer-commitment-code/#questions-answers

Personal Care Products Council. "Member Companies." *About Us*. https://www.personalcarecouncil.org/about-us/member-companies/

Personal Care Products Council. "Home." *Home*. https://www.personalcarecouncil.org/

Prasad, Eswara. *Antioxidants Market by Type (Natural (Vitamin A, Vitamin B, Vitamin C, and Rosemary Extract), Synthetic (Butylated Hydroxyanisole, Butylated Hydroxytoluene, and Others) - Global Opportunity Analysis and Industry Forecast, 2014-2022*. Allied Market Research. (Dec. 2016). https://www.alliedmarketresearch.com/anti-oxidants-market/purchase-options

PR Newswire. "2019 RealSelf Sun Safety Report: Only 1 in 10 Americans Uses Sunscreen Daily; Men Significantly More Likely Than Women to Reapply Sunscreen and Get Annual Skin Check." (July 24, 2019). https://www.prnewswire.com/news-releases/2019-realself-sun-safety-report-only-1-in-10-americans-uses-sunscreen-daily-men-significantly-more-likely-than-women-to-reapply-sunscreen-and-get-annual-skin-check-300889933.html

Purnamawati, Schandra et al. "The Role of Moisturizers in Addressing Various Kinds of Dermatitis: A Review." *Clinical medicine & research* vol. 15,3-4 (2017): 75-87. doi:10.3121/cmr.2017.1363

Ralph's Closet. *Derny's Gay Paree Vanishing Cream Small Bottle Boudoir Vanity Piece 1920s Cosmetics Flapper Logo*. Product. *Pinterest*. https://www.pinterest.ph/pin/829929037559384223/

Randhawa, M., et al. "Daily Use of a Facial Broad-Spectrum Sunscreen Over One-Year Significantly Improves Clinical Evaluation of Photoaging." Dermatol Surg. 2016 Dec;42(12):1354-1361. doi: 10.1097/DSS.00000 00000000879. PMID: 27749441.

Sethi, Anisha et al. "Moisturizers: The Slippery Road." *Indian journal of dermatology* vol. 61,3 (2016): 279-87. doi:10.4103/0019-5154.182427

Sherrow, Victoria. "Encyclopedia of Hair: A Cultural History." *Greenwood Publishing Group,* p.8 (2006). https://books.google.com/books?id=9 Z6vCGbf66YC&pg=PA8&lpg=PA8&dq=radio+ads+shampoo&sou rce=bl&ots=YM4fAZr9ua&sig=ACfU3U2kd9cyThjaMqA1zHDkSv OMKrsXew&hl=en&sa=X&ved=2ahUKEwjl0rvlhPHkAhWNzlkK HfQ9BykQ6AEwCXoECAcQAQ#v=onepage&q=radio%20ads%20 shampoo&f=false

Simpson, Jon. "Finding Brand Success In The Digital World." *Forbes*. (Aug. 25th 2017). https://www.forbes.com/sites/forbesagencycouncil/2017/08/25/ finding-brand-success-in-the-digital-world/#4f4e3f10626e

Tarnopolsky, Mark. "Endurance exercise prevents premature aging: McMaster study." *McMaster University*. Hamilton, Ontario. (Feb 21st 2011). https:// fhs.mcmaster.ca/main/news/news_2011/exercise_and_aging_study.html

Trehan, S., Michniak-Kohn, B., Beri, K. *Plant stem cells in cosmetics: current trends and future directions. Future Sci OA.* 2017;3(4): FSO226. Published 2017 Jul 12. doi:10.4155/fsoa-2017-0026

Vanity Treasures. "Vintage Cosmetic Set / Vintage Cosmetic Sets/Vintage Sample Make-Up Kit /Vintage Sample Make-Up Sample Kits." Product. http://www.vanitytreasures.com/cosmetic_sets_samples/01.htm

Vartan, Starre. *Are You Washing Your Face Too Much?* (Treehugger, Feb. 2020). https://www.treehugger.com/could-the-no-cleanser-experiment-clear -up-your-acne-4868516

Wikipedia contributors. "The Emperor's New Clothes." *Wikipedia, The Free Encyclopedia.* https://en.wikipedia.org/w/index.php?title=The_Emperor%27s_New_Clothes&oldid=939243201

Wikipedia contributors. "Vaseline." *Wikipedia, The Free Encyclopedia.* (Feb 18, 2020) https://en.wikipedia.org/w/index.php?title=Vaseline&oldid=941394564

Williams, J. D., et al. "SPF 100+ sunscreen is more protective against sunburn than SPF 50+ in actual use: Results of a randomized, double-blind, split-face, natural sunlight exposure clinical trial." J Am Acad Dermatol. 2018 May;78(5):902-910.e2. doi: 10.1016/j.jaad.2017.12.062. Epub 2017 Dec 29. PMID: 29291958.

Xu, Suhong, and Andrew D Chisholm. *C. elegans epidermal wounding induces a mitochondrial ROS burst that promotes wound repair. Developmental cell* vol. 31,1 (2014): 48-60. doi:10.1016/j.devcel.2014.08.002

Zhang, Y., et al. Effect of shampoo, conditioner, and permanent waving on the molecular structure of human hair. *PeerJ.* 2015;3:e1296. (Oct 1, 2015). doi:10.7717/peerj.1296

About the Author

Fayne L. Frey, MD is a board-certified dermatologist and skincare consultant, a lover of petroleum jelly, and an avid wrinkle defender. She is a graduate of Weill Cornell Medical College in New York City. Dr. Frey has often been called "The Ralph Nader of the Skincare Industry." For more than three decades, she has clarified marketing claims of advertisers, debunked popular beauty myths, and championed the idea that beauty doesn't come in a bottle.

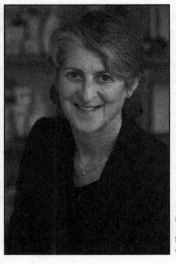

© Shay Frey

She is a regular contributor to the top-rated *50Plus-Today* online magazine. Her articles and medical expertise have been featured on NBC, in *Readers Digest*, *Prevention*, *The Doctor Weighs In*, *Runners World*, *Derm Store*, and many others. She captivates live audiences with her commonsensical approach to skincare and has shared her passion on numerous TV and radio outlets including CBS, Z100 Radio, WOR710 Radio, and various cable networks.

Dr. Frey is the founder of FryFace.com, an educational website that simplifies the overwhelming choice of effective, safe, and affordable products. Her most treasured activities include her daily early-morning five-mile run with friends, playing piano, and spending time in Lake George, New York, with her husband and their four grown children.

Acknowledgments

Writing a book is, unquestionably, one of the most introspective and time-consuming activities one can ever endure. You spend days, weeks, and months, years even, contemplating, doubting yourself, researching, writing, rewriting, doubting yourself some more, editing, reading, and rereading chapters about a subject matter that you're passionate about, even though you may not be exactly sure why. And although you are well aware that very few people around you are as fascinated by the subject matter as you are, for some unknown reason, you are driven to persist.

Writing a book is also an enlightening endeavor. You appreciate the people in your life who put up with your incessant commentary about the book, listen attentively, ask about its progress, express excitement, and encouragement, not necessarily because they're interested in the topic, although some are, but because they're interested in you. I don't know what I did to deserve such supportive people in my life, but I do know how grateful I am for them.

The luckiest day in my life was the day I was born. My mom, a gifted knitter, is the consummate Jewish mother who yearns for nothing more than to have her family together. My dad, a successful businessman, is a principled intellect who loves golf and prefers burnt hot dogs over filet mignon. It is with the deepest of gratitude that I thank my parents, Peggy and Murray Pitkowsky, for urging me to stay true to my convictions, for being the guiding light in my life, and for their endless encouragement with this effort and every other.

I want to thank my sister, Lisa Birch, who braved through hundreds of conversations about the book yet somehow remained the never-ending wind to my back, always making me feel optimistic and empowered. And for reviewing the manuscript as well. To my daughter, Shay, who has been the backbone of my passion, thank you for the hours you spent in front of the computer screen, sharing your creative talents with me, designing the FryFace website, and for touching my heart and the hearts of readers with your manuscript edits. And to all my children, Tali, Shay, Zach, Becca, and Solomon, who have taken time out of their busy lives to express and share with me and others their pride in my pursuits. To my sister, Erica, who I think should've gone into public relations, as she always finds a way to get my message to a larger audience, thank you. To Sheila Bass, my treasured aunt from Texas, "the one who worked for NASA," thank you for believing in me. And to Roger Frey, MD, the hardest working husband and most adoring father, thank you for putting up with me and my strong-willed passions. Life with you is an extraordinary gift and I am ever so grateful.

I want to thank the many professionals for whom without their support completing this project would not have been possible. Thank you to Skyhorse Publishing for taking a chance on this bold writing, and Nicole Mele, for turning my manuscript into a book. Thank you Linda Langton and assistants at

Langtons International Literary Agency for finding a home for *The Skincare Hoax*. Thank you Randy Peyser at AuthorOneStop who has guided me throughout the entire publishing process and introduced me to more amazing people than should be allowed. And to Lana McAra, editor extraordinaire, whose literary skills made my story readable. Thank you to Justin Loeber and his incredible team at MOUTH Digital + Public Relations for helping me expose my message to the masses. And to Jon James and his talented staff at Ignited Results, thank you for building my strong LinkedIn community.

A very special thank you to Patricia Salber, MD, for writing such a meaningful foreword, and giving me a voice on your phenomenal online magazine *The Doctor Weighs In*. Thank you, Leslie Farin, for sharing my articles with your readers at *50plus-Today*, for your fastidious manuscript review, and for endorsing my book. Thank you to Anna Villarreal for our years of collaboration, for sharing our common interest in women's health, for your manuscript review, and also for your endorsement. Thank you to Gay Rodgers, for reviewing the manuscript, for endorsing my book, and for sharing your passion at *Hameua Farm in the Big Valley* with Shay. Thank you, Nancy Parkes, for your boundless encouragement and for your endorsement. The world needs more educators like you. Thank you, Mary Leahy, MD, for your relentless commitment to our community, for your friendship, and for endorsing this book.

To my dearest friends, Debi Ferraris-Teaton, Carol Cosenza, Laura DiMarino, Katie Ottenheimer, and Gelly Neustadt, thank you for being the "sure thing" that I look forward to every single morning. Despite the rain (okay, sometimes my allergies kick in), wind, snow, and even a pandemic, I want to thank you for listening to my habitual lectures as I purged my frustrations during our five mile jaunts. At least those rants made us run faster!

I want to thank the late, award-winning bestselling author, Mary Higgins Clark, the Queen of Suspense, a dear friend who inspired me to write and complete this book. As a first-time author, I asked Mary for some worldly advice as I embarked on this writing journey. Her quick-witted response consisted of three words, "Finish the book." Those words of wisdom resonated with me at every roadblock.

I want to thank the experienced cosmetic chemist, Perry Romanowski, who has shared his expertise with me on numerous occasions.

Thank you, Tracey Damiani, for writing the letter about your experience with the skincare industry and allowing me to share it with my readers. To the extremely bright sister and brother team, Sneha Varghese and Sibin Peter, thank you for sharing your social media and computer talents with me. To Illana Raia, the ultimate optimist, talented author, and friend, thank you for all your worldly advice. And to Gail Cirlin-Lazerus, for taking the time to read my manuscript and for sharing your very helpful insights with me about self-worth.

To my patients, thank you for inspiring me every single day, for sharing your life challenges with me, and for the opportunity to care for you and your skin health. It was through the sharing of your personal struggles with physical flaws that I realized the impact our culture has on most women, and men, too. I am forever grateful. To my loyal and talented office staff, Susan Haimowitz, Jean Santa Teresa, and Adele Tesseyman, thank you for your years of commitment and diligence, and for welcoming our patients every day with a smile. I couldn't do what I do without you.

And to every reader who has taken the time to read this book and started the conversation about real beauty and what's truly important with their family and friends, thank you. Together we can change this narrative, one awesome person at a time.

Index